Bringing a Loved One Home From the Hospital

A How-to Manual for New Caregivers

Dr. Julie Crenshaw

This book is dedicated to all of the caregivers I have met in my years working in home health, and the millions of caregivers who I will never get to meet in person. You are the unsung heros who work tirelessly to care for and advocate for your loved ones. The care you give matters, and you are doing a wonderful job.

With so much love and respect, Julie.

Letter to Caregivers

Dear Caregiver,

Caregiving can be brought on little by little, or all of a sudden. No matter how it comes to you, it can easily reach the point of becoming overwhelming.

You want to make sure your loved one is getting the best care possible, but you might not feel confident about how to make that happen. You can easily feel overwhelmed by the amount of things that need to be done, worried that something important will be missed, and unsure how or when to report your concerns to your loved one's healthcare team.

In my years working in home health, I have spent a LOT of time after a visit standing in the kitchen, on the front porch, or out in the driveway listening to caregivers share with me about their worries and fears, and telling me things they won't say anywhere else. I know the questions you have and frustrations you face, and I'm here to help.

You likely haven't been trained to do this caregiving job, but here you are: doing it around the clock. Let me help answer your questions, ease your stress, and give you some much needed cheerleading along the way! You CAN do this, but you don't have to do it alone.

All my best,

Julie

P.s. Here are some other great resources for you if you'd like to plug into them:

- Join my free facebook group for caregivers:

  - www.facebook.com/groups/caregiversofaginglovedones

- Find me on instagram

  - www.instagram.com/helpthecaregiver

- Learn more about caregiving on my YouTube channel

  - www.youtube.com/@helpthecaregiver

- Send me an email with feedback or questions to

  - julie@helpthecaregiver.com

Contents

Introduction   1

Understanding the Discharge Process   5

  Intensive Care Unit (ICU)

  Acute Care

  Inpatient Rehab

  Skilled Nursing Facility

  Length of Stay Expectations

  Outpatient Therapy

  Home Health

  Palliative Care

  Hospice

  Summary

#1 Following Up with the Doctors   21

  Who Is Their Main Doctor?

  What if They Don't Have a Primary Doctor (PCP)?

  Purpose of Hospital Follow Up Visits

  Did the Hospital Schedule Any Appointments?

  Changing Appointments or Doctors

  Why Are There So Many Appointments?

  Making New Appointments

  Medication & Follow Up Visits

Getting the Most Out of Doctors Appointments

#2 Organizing Medication   37

Why Did My Loved One End Up in the Hospital?

Getting Everything Ready

Finding Out What They Usually Take

Communicating with the Doctor About Problems You Find

Mystery Medication

Medication the Hospital Changed

Keeping Track of Medications

Use the Pharmacist as a Resource

#3 Home Safety   61

Basic Supplies

Getting Into the House

Sleeping Arrangements

Bathroom Safety

Stairs

Floor Coverings

Getting Out of the House

#4 Getting Equipment & Supplies   81

Insurance

Items Ordered by the Hospital

More Insurance Rules

What if the Item Delivered is Not the Right One?

Braces

Lift Chairs

Insurance allowance

What if There is No Insurance, or Insurance Doesn't Cover
Something That is Needed?

Items that Insurance May Not Cover

Hospice Coverage of Medical Supplies

#5 Staying OUT of the Hospital   99

    CABG – "Heart Bypass Surgery"

    CHF -"Heart Failure"

    Heart Attack

    COPD

    Pneumonia

    Orthopedic Surgeries

    Total Hip Replacement

    Total Knee Replacement

    Back Surgery

    Preventing Infection After Surgery

    Blood Clots

    Pain Medication

    UTI – "Urinary Tract Infection"

    Summary

#6 Dizziness   143

    Vertigo

    Dizziness Related to Blood Pressure

    Last Thoughts on Dizziness

#7 Falls   157

    Why Your Loved One is Falling

    A Final Note on Falls

#8 Dividing Responsibilities   165

    Where Will They Stay?

    Who is Taking Care of Medication and Doctor Visits?

    How Are the Bills Getting Paid?

How is the Person Getting to Doctors Appointments and Other Events?

How are Their Daily Living Needs Going to be Met?

How Will They Stay Safe?

Does Someone Need Financial and/or Medical Power of Attorney?

Who Will be the Backup Person if Someone Gets Sick?

#9 Getting the Help You Need   177

Self Care the Right Way

Managing Your Mental Health at Home

Help with Mental Health

Anxiety and Depression

Boosting Mental Health Through Community

Asking for Help from Others

#10 Resources   199

Final Thoughts   205

Master Checklist   206

Acknowledgements   213

About the Author   215

Also By...   217

Introduction

Being a caregiver is a challenging role that few people truly understand. It's a bit like becoming a parent—you can't fully comprehend it until you experience it for yourself, and there's no way to be fully prepared.

I witnessed the caregiving journey firsthand when I watched my grandmother care for my grandfather as his early onset Alzheimer's progressed over a 15-year period. I saw the toll it took on her gradually, until it had affected every area of her life. Witnessing her emotional distress and its negative impact on her health made me very aware of the needs of caregivers I encounter in my work in home health.

Having worked in this field for many years, I found myself repeatedly answering the same questions, making the same phone calls, and providing the same reassurances again and again. It struck me how universal the caregiving experience can be, considering how isolating and lonely it can feel.

Many people have told me that there are no resources for caregivers, and while that's not entirely true, there is definitely a significant gap. Many available resources are relatively unknown, and few provide practical education or training.

Caregiving is complex, and certain aspects are very time-sensitive. Many caregivers I encounter in my work are new to the role or relatively new, feeling frantic and overwhelmed as they try to navigate everything all at once.

For many people, caregiving seems to be thrown on them without warning. A loved one may have experienced a medical emergency or an accident that created an instant change from independent living to needing around the clock care, requiring a ton of resources and numerous medical appointments.

This book is for you if you're new to caregiving or have been in the role for some time but still feel confused and overwhelmed about how to best care for your loved one. Maybe you're fairly comfortable in your caregiving role but never received proper education or training and want to make sure you're covering all your bases.

Are you currently in a situation where your loved one is in the hospital, and you're desperately searching for answers about how to prepare for their discharge, whether it's to their own house or yours? Friend, this book is exactly what you need!

In this book, I'll address the top 10 issues that I see new caregivers commonly face. These are the issues that often cause anxiety and overwhelm, and if not addressed quickly, can sometimes lead to the person ending up back in the hospital - which is the last thing anyone wants!

I'll address these issues in order of importance, which means tackling the most time-sensitive concerns first. If you have a specific worry causing you stress, feel free to jump to that section. However, please understand that **the chapters on following up with the doctor, organizing medication, home safety, and staying out of the hospital should be read as soon as possible to ensure safety and minimize the chance of your loved one returning to the hospital.**

There is a wealth of information in this book, and I've made every effort to make it easy to read and easy to put into action. Throughout the book, you'll find stopping points to reflect on what you've learned and identify the next steps you need to take.

At the end of the book, you'll find a master checklist covering every item we've gone over. If you prefer a printable checklist that you can physically write on, visit www.helpthecaregiver.com/home-from-the-hospital-chec klist to get your printable master checklist today!

I understand that this can feel overwhelming, and like you have a million things to do, but please don't let yourself become consumed by it all. This book was created specifically for you, and we'll get through this together! Start from the beginning, use the checklists to write down notes about what to do next, and take it one section at a time.

Safety is our top priority. Let's ensure your loved one is safe and stable while providing you with the resources you need. Ready? Let's get started!

Understanding the Discharge Process

B efore we dive into what to do after a person leaves the hospital, let's talk a bit about the different types of places they can go. I've seen so many cases where patients come straight home from the hospital and the caregiver feels upset or frustrated that they didn't go somewhere else first for "rehab."

It's really helpful to understand what these different places are, and who is best suited for them. That way, you can feel more confident about how your situation was handled.

When I first graduated from physical therapy school, I was hired to work for a hospital system. It was a great job, especially right out of school, because I was able to work in a variety of settings and gain a lot of experience. I still had all the information fresh in my mind from grad school, and this setting reinforced all of that new knowledge.

Sometimes, I would work on the acute care floor at the hospital, and that's where I want to start our discussion about different settings. If someone has a medical emergency, they usually end up in the hospital. They stay in the "acute care" department, which is meant to be a short-term stay. The person has a medical issue that needs a lot of attention, but they are expected to get better within a few days. In really serious cases, they might go to the intensive care unit (ICU) first to be stabilized, and then they'll be moved to the acute floor for further monitoring.

Once the person is medically stable and getting ready for discharge, we have to think about where they need to go next. The hospital's main concern at that point is the person's safety. Can they go home and take care of themselves without any problems? If not, what kind of help do they need? What level of support is best for them?

As a physical therapist, it was my job to figure out the answers to these questions when I worked on the acute care floor. I had to recommend the most suitable place for patients based on their physical abilities, stamina, and the support they had from caregivers.

Let's go over the main healthcare settings and what you can expect from them in terms of medical care and therapy.

Intensive Care Unit (ICU)

This is where the most sick and unstable patients go. They're more likely to have a downturn in their condition and need immediate medical care while they're in the hospital. The staff keeps a close eye on them and takes extra precautions, like wearing extra protective gear, because they're at a higher risk of complications.

Patients in the ICU might or might not receive therapy while they're there. Some patients are too sick to participate, and it's actually not in their best interest to push them when they're medically unstable. Resting and stabilizing their bodies, even if it means getting physically weaker, takes priority. Overexerting themselves could worsen their condition instead of improving it.

However, there are patients who need close monitoring but are stable enough to engage in basic therapy. This helps them maintain their strength or gives them a boost for recovery. The decision about whether a patient can participate in therapy is made by the treating team.

In the ICU, therapy sessions are usually short, around 15 minutes. They focus on basic movements like rolling in bed, sitting up while maintaining balance, standing at the edge of the bed, or taking a few steps in the room. It may not seem like much, but it's a big task for these patients.

Therapy is most commonly provided to patients who are generally stable and being prepared to move from the ICU to the acute care floor. It helps them demonstrate their strength and stability, showing that they no longer require ICU-level care.

Acute Care

Most patients on the acute floor don't need extensive physical therapy during their stay. Typically, they're expected to be there for only a few days. In this setting, physical therapy primarily assesses the patient's current physical condition and determines the next steps. Some patients who received physical therapy in the ICU may require more therapy involvement on the acute care floor.

These patients still need close monitoring by the nursing staff and doctors, so therapy isn't the main focus. It may involve basic exercises while sitting on the edge of the bed or gradually building endurance by walking in their room or the hallway.

If a patient just underwent surgery, therapy makes sure they're aware of any surgical precautions. They help with getting the patient up and check for any bad reactions to the surgery that might require an extended hospital stay, such as fainting or getting very dizzy when they stand, or unusually high pain during movement.

Certain hospitals have specialized areas specifically for routine orthopedic surgeries. In these cases, therapy may be more involved in the postsurgical care before the patient is discharged. Again, this therapy isn't meant to be intense. Its purpose is to make sure the patient is recovering normally, provide instructions about precautions, and help the patient perform the expected postsurgical exercises.

Most patients who are admitted to the hospital can go home without needing additional help. They received the right care to address the problem that brought them to the hospital, and they're feeling much better; ready to rest for a few days and return to their normal routine.

However, there are many patients who can't simply go home and take care of themselves. These patients may already have ongoing medical issues that require assistance. Or, they might have experienced a significant medical event like a severe stroke, heart attack, or accident resulting in multiple broken bones, causing them to be unable to care for themselves even if they could before being hospitalized.

If it's determined that the patient is physically unable to care for themselves at home without assistance, it becomes the hospital staff's responsibility to decide the most suitable alternative. Let's discuss the most common options in these cases.

Inpatient Rehab

Inpatient rehab can be summed up in one word: intense! When speaking with families whose loved ones were sent home with home health services, many times they will express frustration that their loved one wasn't sent to inpatient rehab first. I'm often surprised by this, considering what I see from my clinical perspective about what their loved one can tolerate.

I want to help families understand the typical inpatient rehab experience, so let me take a moment to explain it here. Many people genuinely benefit from inpatient rehab, and I have so much respect for my colleagues working in this setting. They are absolutely amazing, doing the heavy lifting that most people simply wouldn't have the ability to do, day in and day out.

The standard expectation in inpatient rehab is that a person will undergo three hours of therapy every single day, six days a week! Yes, you read that right. Three hours a day. The amount of therapy time can be divided among the different disciplines based on the patient's needs, and it doesn't have to be evenly distributed.

For instance, if a patient requires only physical therapy, they would complete three hours of physical therapy daily. If they need both physical therapy and occupational therapy, they might do an hour and a half of each, or maybe one hour of one therapy and two hours of the other. It depends on their specific needs.

When a caregiver tells me how upset they are that they feel their feeble 85-year-old mother was wronged by not being sent to inpatient rehab, I want to make sure they understand why that decision was absolutely the right one. Their poor mother would never be able to handle three hours of therapy each day, and it would be terrible to push her so hard. Personally, if I spent 3 hours at the gym, I'd be exhausted! There are better ways to get this patient the care she needs.

During my time at the hospital, I also worked in the inpatient rehab unit. I hated the times when I found myself apologizing repeatedly to patients who expressed exhaustion and felt they couldn't continue with therapy for the day. I couldn't let them to return to bed yet because they hadn't met their required therapy minutes for the day, so we had to keep pushing and pushing to make sure they weren't forced to discharge early.

To be clear, if a person is unable to meet the expected amount of therapy in inpatient rehab, they will be discharged. Insurance closely monitors this situation and may request the rehab unit to discharge the patient if the time requirements are not being met. There's no point in sending them to rehab if they don't have the stamina for that level of therapy. Those spots should be reserved for individuals who can benefit the most from it.

Skilled Nursing Facility

A skilled nursing facility is a great option when a patient needs significant assistance with personal care, and can engage in a good amount of daily therapy, but needs less intensity than would be required in inpatient rehab.

That's not to say skilled nursing is easy, because it's not! Although the therapy expectations are lower, patients still spend about an hour and a half on therapy daily. Again, this time can be divided between different therapy disciplines, but it's still a lot.

There are still many patients I encounter who wouldn't be able to handle that much therapy. And again, if they can't consistently participate in the required therapy, they will be discharged quickly because the insurance will require it.

A few things to note about skilled nursing facilities: Sometimes the presence or absence of a caregiver can determine whether a person is sent to skilled nursing or not. Patients who might otherwise be able to go home because their condition is expected to improve and their recovery is easier may be sent to rehab if they lack a caregiver to help with their daily needs or handle emergencies outside the home.

Sometimes a patient may not be an ideal candidate for skilled nursing because it would be too physically demanding for them. However, their caregiver has indicated that they won't be able to provide care until the patient gets stronger. This can be the case when the caregiver has their own medical issues, an older spouse who can't lift their partner, or an adult child who works during the day and needs the patient's basic needs to be managed while they're away. These situations can be tricky, and every case is different.

Another important aspect of skilled nursing facilities is that, although there is plenty of staff available to care for patients, it's expected that patients are medically stable. While there is a supervising doctor at the facility who oversees patient care, they typically won't make rounds or have face-to-face interactions with the patients during their stay. There may be exceptions if a person has a change in their medical status after going to the skilled nursing facility, but the standard practice is that nurses will be available to give medication and monitor the patients. It is not expected that the doctor will be actively treating them.

I often encounter individuals who believe their loved one should have been seen by a doctor while at the skilled nursing facility, so I want to clarify that it's not a standard practice during their stay. The staff assists with personal care, medication administration, and meal delivery, but patients are expected to be well enough not to require a doctor's visit while there.

Length of Stay Expectations

As we mentioned earlier, an acute care stay typically lasts only a few days. Of course, there are exceptions, but in general, most patients spend less than a week on the acute care floor.

The ICU is a different story. Patients remain there until they are stable, and that's the primary factor determining their length of stay.

Both inpatient rehab and skilled nursing facilities have an average length of stay of 21 days. Occasionally, a person may stay for a week longer, but it's relatively rare and requires extensive paperwork and approvals.

In recent years, insurance companies have implemented a system of reimbursement based on the patient's reason for being in the facility. The aim is to provide appropriate and necessary care without prolonging stays unnecessarily. When a person is admitted to inpatient rehab or a skilled nursing facility, there needs to be a single primary reason listed for their stay. After determining the primary reason, the staff, including nurses and therapists, do their best to paint a more complete picture of the patient and identify other factors that may affect their recovery time.

For example, if we consider a 35-year-old man who was working full-time before being hospitalized due to a severe car accident that resulted in multiple fractures, we would expect him to regain his strength and mobility within a fairly short timeframe.

On the other hand, if we have an 80-year-old woman who suffered a stroke and has other medical issues like heart failure and COPD, we would expect a slower recovery. The newer insurance calculations attempt to account for these differences and would generally approve a slightly longer stay for the older woman compared to the younger man.

With all that said, it's important to note that a 21-day stay is not guaranteed for everyone, but it serves as the expected maximum length of time for most patients. This is a point I often discuss with caregivers because many assume that a patient will stay in these settings until they're 100% better, but that's not the case.

The goal of these facilities is to help patients become strong, stable, and safe enough to return home. It's not meant to be a place for them to stay until they have fully recovered. That's where outpatient therapy and home health come into play. Let's take a moment to discuss those settings.

Outpatient Therapy

There are many reasons why someone might be referred to outpatient therapy. Having worked in outpatient therapy myself, I can confidently list many great benefits of this incredible setting. Outpatient therapists are like the wizards of the therapy world. They have access to all the fancy therapy gadgets, fun machines, and a wide array of amazing techniques they use to provide hands-on care for various pains and problems.

In an outpatient facility, the general expectation is that a person will complete an average of one hour of therapy per session, typically 2 to 3 times a week, and they will be working hard during each session. Depending on the reason for referral, a typical amount of time spent in outpatient could be anywhere from 4 to 12 weeks, with a more typical average of 6 to 8 weeks.

Patients are often discharged from the hospital directly to outpatient therapy for various reasons. For instance, they may have undergone orthopedic surgery like hip, knee, or shoulder replacement. Others may require cardiac rehab following a heart attack, or they may have experienced a stroke or other injury that significantly impacted their physical abilities. Typically, these patients are on the younger side (65 or less) and were relatively healthy before their hospital admission.

Another great advantage of outpatient therapy is the opportunity to get out of the house. It can do wonders for a person's motivation to leave their home and actively work towards their recovery in a therapy setting.

Many patients I work with in home health struggle with anxiety and depression because they are confined to their homes, rarely experiencing anything beyond their four walls. Going through the process of getting ready, leaving the house, and participating in physical therapy outside their home can have a great positive impact on their mental health.

However, there are situations where it may not be possible or feasible to access outpatient therapy.

Home Health

Home health services are designed to cater to patients who are unable to go to other settings. To qualify for home health, a patient must be considered "homebound." It's important to clarify that being homebound doesn't mean the person is completely unable to leave their house. Instead, it signifies that leaving the home requires a "taxing effort."

Examples of a "taxing effort" can include needing assistance from another person to leave the house due to driving limitations or the need to transport medical equipment (like a walker) for mobility. It can also involve relying on a wheelchair due to difficulties with mobility, making it physically challenging to enter and exit the house. Limited energy is another factor, such as needing to rest or nap for the remainder of the day after a short trip to the grocery store.

The general expectation for patients receiving home health services is that they do not leave their homes except for essential trips such as medical appointments, worship services, or short grocery trips. The majority of their time is spent at home, primarily due to medical necessity rather than personal preference.

An example of a great candidate for home health is an older patient with heart and breathing issues who underwent back surgery and requires physical therapy. However, this individual cannot tolerate going to outpatient therapy due to the energy-draining process of getting out of bed, getting dressed, leaving the house, and commuting to the outpatient office. By having the physical therapist come to their house, all their energy can be focused on the therapy session rather than the exhausting preparations and commute.

Another example could be a patient who has experienced a sickness or medical emergency, such as a stroke or heart attack, resulting in significant weakness and multiple medical issues that limit their ability to handle several hours of therapy per day. Although they need therapy, they would be unable to meet the requirements of inpatient rehab or a skilled nursing facility, and they don't have the ability to get to an outpatient facility multiple times a week. Home health allows them to receive therapy at a slower pace and over a longer duration.

Home health is also very beneficial for patients who need multiple types of therapy that are not always available in outpatient (such as speech therapy), and/or who need ongoing nursing care.

While inpatient rehab and skilled nursing facilities typically have a maximum three-week stay expectation, home health services are usually provided for at least two months or even longer. One exception to this timeframe is patients who have undergone surgery and need a few weeks to build up strength and manage pain before transitioning to outpatient therapy.

Being able to safely get in and out of the house can also play a role in the choice of home health services. Some individuals have houses with stairs that pose challenges due to pain and weakness. In these cases, home health may be used for a few weeks to help the patient strengthen and navigate the stairs safely before transitioning to outpatient therapy.

Palliative Care

I want to use this section to also explain a little bit more about palliative and hospice care, because so little is known about these services, and there are a lot of misunderstandings about their purpose and how they work. With both of these services, information is free with no obligation to agree to services, so please don't hesitate to reach out to a local provider with questions.

Palliative care is focused on providing relief from diseases or serious illnesses such as cancer, dementia, lung disease, kidney failure, Parkinson's disease, cystic fibrosis, end-stage liver disease, etc. It addresses symptoms such as pain, nausea, anxiety, loss of appetite, fatigue, and trouble sleeping, among other things. The palliative care team includes doctors, nurses, chaplains, social workers, and nutritionists. Palliative care can be paired WITH other services for more comprehensive help for the patient. You can have palliative care AND home health. You can have palliative care AND continue to take ongoing treatments for diseases such as cancer, with the aim of full recovery.

If your loved one's pain or symptoms don't seem to be managed well enough with the care they are currently getting, you might see if adding palliative care could help to provide relief and support. There are resources with more information about palliative care in the resources chapter.

Hospice

Hospice care is very different than it was a few decades ago. Unfortunately, many people are scared to even say the word "hospice," much less have a conversation about it, because there is a lot of confusion and outdated information about what hospice is and how it works. I also want to say up front that different hospice companies have different policies, so if you get answers you don't like from the first company you speak with, reach out to another one to see if they are more aligned with your loved one's needs.

Let's get a few myths out of the way up front:

Myth #1: Going on hospice does not mean that the person is about to die. It means that the person has a disease or illness that they are not expected to recover from, such as end-stage kidney disease. I've known many patients who were on hospice services for a year or longer, and I've also known patients who transitioned to hospice while they went through intense cancer treatment that took everything out of them, and then when they went into remission and started feeling stronger, they transitioned back to home health to continue with a full recovery.

Myth #2: Hospice will not take all the person's medication from them. They may cover an off-brand version instead of the name brand version (because hospice pays for all of a patient's medication when they come on services), and there may be some medications that are not covered under hospice, but for the most part, the person's medication routine should not change. This is definitely something to ask about before signing up for hospice, because there are exceptions, but it's not the same as it was several decades ago when medications were all stopped.

Myth #3: Hospice is not going to speed up a person's death by giving them unlimited amounts of morphine. I know this is also a big fear among many of my patients and their caregivers. Hospice is a comfort service, and their goal is to keep the patient comfortable, but only within the limits discussed with and agreed on by the patient and their family. They will not medicate a patient without informed consent of the patient and/or family.

Fact #1: Hospice will pay for all of the needs of a patient in their care. This includes major medical equipment (like a hospital bed or bedside commode), medication, personal care supplies, such as adult diapers, barrier creams for the person's bottom, and bed pads.

Fact #2: You cannot get therapy services while on hospice. Hospice is considered a comfort service, not a restorative service, so physical, occupational, and speech therapy services are not covered except in extreme circumstances. I have seen a few patients on hospice who received home health therapy for a short time after falling and breaking a hip or having an extreme downturn in their physical strength after a major medical problem. If your loved one needs hospice, but might benefit from therapy services to establish an exercise program, or for caregiver training to help with physically moving the patient in bed or transferring them to a wheelchair, have home health come in for a short time (maybe a month), and then transition to hospice services.

Fact #3: Someone can come to your home to talk about hospice and answer all of your questions about medication, other medical treatments, what equipment can be covered, and how often they will come out. This is a free visit with no obligation to sign up for services. If it doesn't feel like a good fit, say no or reach out to a different company. Tell that company what you didn't like about the answers you got from the first company and ask if they do things differently. Keep going until you find an answer that feels good to you.

Summary

The purpose of this section was to help you understand the different settings available for individuals to recover after a medical event, as well as the considerations made by the medical staff when recommending a particular setting.

Key factors in this decision include the patient's medical stability, required care (nursing, therapy, wound care), safety at home, expected length of recovery, and their ability to tolerate the therapy required in inpatient rehab or skilled nursing facilities.

The medical team will be asking and reporting on all of the following:

1. Is the patient medically stable?

2. What kind of care do they need now? Nursing? Therapy? Wound care?

3. Are they safe to go home? Will they be able to physically get in/out of their house in an emergency? How will they get food? Can they manage their own medications? Do they need help going to the bathroom? Do they have someone who can help them with these things if they can't do it for themselves?

4. How long is it going to take for them to get better? Can they make a lot of progress in a short period of time? Or will their recovery be a slow one?

5. Can they tolerate the required amount of therapy they would need to participate in if we sent them to inpatient rehab or a skilled nursing facility?

My aim is for you to have a better understanding of the journey your loved one may have gone through before coming into your care. I also hope that if another hospitalization happens, you will be better equipped with knowledge about available options and how the process works.

Now You Know:

- The different therapy expectations in different settings

- The standard length of stay expected in different settings

- The many considerations the hospital team took into account when recommending which setting was best for your loved one

Now that your loved one is under your care, I want you to feel confident about your ability to meet their needs, and to help minimize any anxiety that may come with taking on this new caregiver role.

Let's dive into the top 10 issues I see caregivers face after bringing a loved one home from the hospital.

#1 Following Up with the Doctors

L et's discuss doctor's appointments. If your loved one has been admitted to the hospital due to a serious medical issue, it's highly likely that they need to follow up with at least one doctor after being discharged home.

Making and prioritizing these appointments should be your first task once you're back home, and it shouldn't take too long if you follow the suggestions here.

There are two big reasons why this is so important and needs to be at the top of your priority list. First, it's very rare for your loved one's doctors to be informed about their hospitalization. Hospitals simply don't have the time or resources to track down all the relevant doctors and provide updates.

Apart from the logistical challenges this would present for the hospital, people frequently change doctors, and there's no guarantee that the doctors listed for your loved one are the most up-to-date. Sending updates to previous doctors you're no longer using would be a HIPAA violation.

Unfortunately, many people either assume that their doctor has been informed about the situation, or they are too caught up in managing the stress of the hospitalization that it doesn't cross their mind that the doctors responsible for their loved one's care are completely unaware of what happened.

Doctors can't address a problem they don't know exists. They also can't adjust treatment if they're unaware of changes in the patient's condition or issues with their medications. So, it's incredibly important to schedule and keep follow-up appointments with any relevant doctors after a hospitalization.

Who Is Their Main Doctor?

Let's break it down further to avoid confusion. Most individuals have a doctor they see for regular check-ups, and there are different terms to refer to this doctor, all essentially meaning the same thing. This doctor might be called:

"Family doctor" - This is an older term used by many patients, referring back to a time when a single doctor would treat the entire family, before the widespread use of specialists. Knowing this term is helpful, especially for individuals from the boomer or silent generation who may not understand which doctor you're referring to otherwise.

"GP" - Short for "general practitioner," this is a doctor who serves as a generalist. Their role involves having a broad knowledge of various medical areas, and they are typically the first point of contact for basic healthcare needs such as check-ups, minor illnesses, and referrals to specialists if necessary.

"PCP" - Abbreviation for "primary care physician." This term refers to the doctor as the primary point of contact when you have a health issue. It became a popular term when insurance companies started requiring referrals to see specialists. Under this care model, the primary doctor is aware of everyone on the patient's care team and coordinates all referrals.

The aim is to have one central person who is familiar with all your needs and the specialists involved in your care.

"Internist" is another term that many people use to describe a primary care physician, although primary doctors can have various specialties, "internal medicine" being one of them. Many primary doctors are trained as internists, so it's become another synonymous term that someone might use when referring to their main doctor.

Throughout the remainder of this book, I'll use the term PCP for simplicity, but you'll understand that I'm referring to the "main" doctor your loved one sees, whether they call them their family doctor, GP, internist, or any other similar term.

I want to note that some individuals use a specialist as their "primary doctor." For instance, a patient with Stage 4 Parkinson's disease but no other major medical conditions may have a neurologist as their primary doctor. While less common, I've encountered many patients whose first point of contact for any health issue is a specialist because they have severe medical problems specific to one specialty area.

I've observed this with patients who have undergone transplants, have advanced-stage cancer, require dialysis, or have bone diseases. **If this applies to your loved one, when I use the term PCP, I'm referring to that specialist who is acting as their primary doctor.**

What if They Don't Have a Primary Doctor (PCP)?

It is incredibly important for your loved one to have a PCP. They need to have someone who is familiar with their personal and family medical history, and someone who can maintain their care, order follow up testing, and write medication refills so that the hospital doesn't become the go-to solution for every question or concerning symptom.

Getting set up with a new primary doctor is as simple as calling the doctor's office and asking to be set up as a new patient. The two main difficulties in getting set up with a preferred doctor is 1) if that doctor is currently accepting new patients (not all doctors have room to take on new patients) and 2) if they accept your loved one's insurance. Some doctors will accept patients as "self pay" if they don't have insurance, and others won't. You won't know until you ask.

To start your search, it's a good idea to call the insurance company and get a list of local in-network doctors to choose from. If the doctor is in-network, all of the costs of using that doctor will be less, because the insurance company will pay more of the bill. There is also less likelihood that the insurance company will deny claims, because you will be using one of their preferred doctors.

Beyond looking at a list and picking someone at random, see if you can ask around locally to get an idea of what people's experience has been with that doctor, and whether or not they would recommend them. Sometimes you can find reviews for the doctor online. Be sure to ask or pay attention to WHY someone does or doesn't like that doctor, because not all people value the same thing in a doctor. Just because they are a good fit for one person, doesn't mean they will be a good fit for your loved one.

Once you have someone picked out, call the office and ask if they can take on your loved one as a new patient. It's important to mention if they've been in the hospital lately and will need follow up care from the hospitalization. If your loved one has seen other doctors in the past, it will be helpful to call those offices and request that the patient's records be sent to the new doctor so that the new doctor can have a more complete understanding of your loved one's medical history.

If this information is not available, it's a good idea to have as much information ready to give as possible about their history medical conditions, surgeries (and dates of surgeries), vaccine history, allergies, current medications, hospitalization history, and family medical history. There is room to record all of this in my log book, "Keep Up with Your Loved One's Doctors All in One." Check it out on my website, www.helpthecaregiver .com/store.

Purpose of Hospital Follow Up Visits

Alright, now that we've clarified what a PCP is, let's discuss the importance of scheduling a follow-up appointment with their PCP after a hospitalization. This visit is known as "hospital follow-up." It's important to inform the PCP about the hospitalization because they should have the most comprehensive understanding of the patient's medical history. Without knowledge of major events like hospitalizations, they cannot provide the best possible care because they lack important information.

What is the purpose of this visit? Here's what you need to accomplish at this visit:

1. Inform the PCP about the hospitalization and give them a copy of the discharge papers if possible.

2. Discuss the reason or possible reasons for the hospitalization, including which body system experienced complications and why (heart, lungs, kidneys, etc). This information will be added to the patient's medical record.

3. Obtain a referral to a new specialist if necessary.

4. Review any medication changes made during the hospitalization. Adjust the patient's records accordingly or have a conversation about what medication to take going forward (more details on this in the next chapter about medications).

5. Conduct a physical examination of the patient post-discharge to confirm their medical stability and expected recovery progress. The PCP may provide additional suggestions to help in their recovery.

6. Address any questions you may have about the patient's health, hospitalization, and recovery.

Did the Hospital Schedule Any Appointments?

Your loved one should have received discharge papers from the hospital when they were discharged. These papers provide a general summary of instructions to follow once they're back home. They may contain a lot of information, including instructions related to specific illnesses or medications for your loved one. If they underwent surgery, the surgeon may have included instructions for post-operative care.

Take a moment to locate those discharge papers and review them to see if there is any information about follow-up appointments with a doctor. Some hospitals may even schedule appointments for a patient before they leave. Otherwise, the papers may simply instruct you to follow up with your doctor once you're back home.

What does the information on the discharge papers say? Are there any appointments already scheduled for the patient after discharge? If so, let's start by reviewing those appointments. Make a note of all the appointments that have been made, whether by writing them down separately, highlighting, or underlining the relevant information.

Changing Appointments or Doctors

If the hospital has already scheduled appointments for the patient, let's focus on those first. **Please note that you are allowed to change these appointments if needed!** If the scheduled appointments don't work with your schedule, call that doctor's office and let them know, "I have an appointment that was made by the hospital, but I need to reschedule it to a different day." They will help you reschedule and find a day and time that works better for you.

If the hospital has made appointments for the patient, you may already know the doctor, or it could be a referral to a new doctor. If you're unfamiliar with the doctor, you have the option to either keep the appointment as scheduled or request a referral to a different doctor. For example, if your loved one was admitted to the hospital due to a new heart issue and they've been referred to a local cardiologist who neither of you know, but you already have a cardiologist who you trust and have been seeing for years, you and your loved one may prefer that they see the doctor you're already familiar with.

If this is the case, the first step I recommend is calling the office of the doctor you'd like your loved one to see (in this example, the cardiologist) and explain, "I've been a patient of Dr. So-and-so's for (however many) years, and my (mom) was just admitted to (local hospital) for (heart problem). They referred her to someone we're not familiar with, and I'd prefer her to be seen by (the doctor's office you're calling). Is he/she currently accepting new patients?"

It's important to make this call first because not all doctors are always accepting new patients. They have limited capacity to see patients each day, and sometimes their patient list is too full to be able to take on new patients. Additionally, some offices that have limited availability to take on new patients may have a policy of only accepting new patients if they are related to an existing patient. That's why it's important to mention that you're a current patient when making the call and explaining the situation regarding your family member.

If the preferred doctor is unable to accept new patients, you have the choice to stick with the original referral or do some research to find another doctor you'd prefer your loved one to see. While it's easier to stick with the referral and the appointment that has already been made, I want you to be aware of your options so that you can make an informed decision about their care. If it doesn't matter to you, or if you've already heard positive things about the referred doctor, then by all means, just go to that appointment!

Keep in mind that some offices may have policies against allowing patients to switch from one doctor within the practice to another. So, it's important to make an effort to be seen by a doctor you feel confident you will want to stay with, because it can sometimes be more challenging to switch later on.

If you want your loved one to see a different doctor than the one they were originally referred to, you'll need to get a new referral from another doctor. The hospital won't be involved in changing the referral for you. However, if you catch this before leaving the hospital, you can request a change in the referral before completing the discharge process. After that, you'll need to handle it outside of the hospital.

Here's what you should do: inform your PCP during the visit that you would like to be referred to a different doctor. You can say, "the hospital referred us to (this cardiologist), but we would like to be referred to (this other cardiologist) instead. Will you please send a referral to the other cardiologist?" Make sure to make this request during the visit with your PCP, because they usually won't do it over the phone if they haven't seen the patient since the hospitalization.

How can you research new doctors to find one you think is a good fit? Research specialists the same way I suggested to find a PCP who would be a good match in the section above, "What if They Don't Have a Primary Doctor (PCP)?" Call the insurance to find out who is in-network. See if you can find reviews online or by asking around for recommendations.

Why Are There So Many Appointments?

Now, let's discuss understanding the referrals made by the hospital. It's not uncommon for patients to receive a list of multiple appointments after a hospital stay, including both familiar and unfamiliar doctors. This can cause anxiety if they're unsure why they have so many doctors to see.

In these cases, I often sit with the patient and help them call each of the new doctor's offices on the list to ask two clarifying questions: 1) What type of doctor is this? (neurologist, cardiologist, orthopedic, etc.), and 2) Can you please tell me why the patient was referred to this office?

It's important to remember that the person answering the phone is not a doctor and doesn't have access to the patient's hospital records. They will likely only be able to see the diagnosis listed on the referral form. They should be able to tell you which diagnosis caused the referral, such as afib, heart failure, stroke management, or follow-up from hip surgery.

The purpose of this call is not to get long answers but to understand the basics of why the referral was sent (e.g., "Okay, this is a heart doctor. They want the patient to follow up with them since they went to the emergency room with chest pain, etc.").

Making New Appointments

Now, let's discuss what to do if the hospital didn't make any appointments for your loved one before discharge. In this case, it's up to you to proactively reach out to the appropriate doctor's offices to schedule any necessary appointments.

I highly recommend prioritizing an appointment with your loved one's PCP. This appointment should be non-negotiable. The PCP is supposed to be the first point of contact, the person who knows the most about your loved one, and the one who can be the patient's strongest advocate on their healthcare journey—but only if they are kept in the loop!

They can't advocate for the patient if they don't know their needs, and they can't provide the best care if they don't know the full story of what's going on. To be frank, most PCPs aren't able to spend a significant amount of time trying to untangle a backlog of six hospital visits since the last time they were informed about their patient's situation in order to create the best plan moving forward.

PCPs that have been treating your loved one for many years may be able to provide more accurate, and faster, treatment for your loved one if they are communicated with as soon as possible. They know so much about their medical history, including past treatments that were not effective or had bad reactions.

They may have a more informed idea of why the hospitalization occurred in the first place, and how to keep them from ending up back in the hospital, but ONLY if they know what's going on in time to help.

It's important to understand how vital the PCP is in helping your loved one have the best outcome possible, so prioritize seeing them within 2 weeks (maximum) of discharge, every single time a hospitalization occurs.

I'll provide an exception here: if your loved one has had multiple back-to-back hospitalizations, you might not be able to get them to the doctor before they end up back in the hospital. I sincerely hope that doesn't happen to you or your loved one, but I see it frequently in home health.

In this case, I still strongly recommend keeping the primary care doctor aware of the situation, even if you have to communicate through different means like an online patient portal or leaving a message for the doctor's nurse. As soon as things are settled and your loved one is truly stable at home, I urge you to make an appointment to update the doctor on everything that has happened since the last visit.

If you're unsure about whether or not there is a need for follow-up appointments with your loved one's specialists, you can wait and discuss your concerns and options with the PCP during that visit. However, you're also welcome to make any necessary appointments to specialists your loved one already sees related to the hospitalization if you feel they are necessary.

For example, if your loved one was hospitalized for a heart problem and already sees a cardiologist, I encourage you to follow up with the cardiologist. The same applies to stroke and a neurologist, or a UTI that requires hospitalization when your loved one already sees a urologist. If your loved one had an accident resulting in bone fractures that required surgery, they will definitely need to follow up with the orthopedic surgeon.

To make the appointment with the specialist, simply call their office and inform them, "(patient's name) is a patient of Dr. So-and-so and they were recently in the hospital for (reason). I would like to schedule an appointment for a hospital follow-up."

Make sure you have a general idea of why you want to come in for the visit in case they ask. Don't get defensive about this! They usually need to input a reason or visit code into the computer to explain the type of visit and any patient requests. They also ask for clarification in order to schedule enough time for the appointment and code it correctly on the schedule for billing and other purposes.

Medication & Follow Up Visits

It's perfectly acceptable to mention that you want to discuss medications that were changed at the hospital, concerning symptoms your loved one has been experiencing, or that you would like the specialist to review the medications they have prescribed for the patient since that was the reason for the hospitalization.

We will cover medications in detail in the upcoming section, but I want to address them in the context of these follow-up visits. Medication miscommunication happens all too often and is a frequent cause of emergency room visits, hospitalizations, and unwanted symptoms or side effects.

I have seen many instances when a hospitalization can trigger medication miscommunication because doctors at the hospital often change a patient's medications. Patients typically receive prescriptions from multiple doctors and specialists, and the hospital doesn't directly communicate these changes to them.

If you don't inform your doctors and specialists about medication changes you were instructed to make, they will assume that you're still taking the medications as previously prescribed. This creates confusion and inaccurate medical records.

Please read the medication section for more insight and specific suggestions on managing potential problems that may come up. However, I want to emphasize the importance of discussing medications during these follow-up visits.

Getting the Most Out of Doctors Appointments

Here are my suggestions to prepare for an MD visit to make sure all the bases have been covered. I want you to feel confident walking into the appointment and not realize afterward that you forgot something important.

- Take all your loved one's medicines to the appointment, or at least an updated list of the medicines, including the dosage and frequency of use.

- Take the discharge paperwork from the hospital, because this paperwork should list any suggested medication changes, which will help with clear communication

- Create a list of questions you want to ask during the appointment, including questions about medications, symptoms, referrals to other doctors, and any necessary resources.

- Bring this list with you and make sure there's enough space to write down all the answers. Don't rely on your memory!

- If you're monitoring your loved one's vital signs (oxygen, heart rate, blood pressure, etc.), bring this information with you as well.

Bonus tips:
- Leave the list of appointment questions somewhere easy to get to in the days leading up to the appointment. Every time you think of something you want to ask, write it down on the list. This will help make sure you remember all the questions you meant to ask when the time comes.

- If there's any concern about your loved one's vital signs, particularly blood pressure, I strongly recommend tracking them for at least a week before the appointment, if possible.

The blood pressure reading at the doctor's appointment can sometimes be higher than normal for several reasons. If you don't have other measurements to refer to, the doctor will make decisions about blood pressure medications based on these infrequent appointments, which can lead to medication-related problems. For more details on this, please refer to the chapters on troubleshooting dizziness and falls.

As a caregiver, being prepared and confident is important for managing your loved one's health effectively. That's why I created two log books to help you on this journey: "Track Your Loved One's Vital Signs" and "Keep Up with Your Loved One's Doctors All in One". These essential resources will empower you with the tools you need for a successful caregiving journey.

The "Track Your Loved One's Vital Signs" log book allows you to track and record vital measurements like blood pressure, heart rate, temperature, weight, oxygen, and blood sugar. By monitoring these regularly, you'll have a comprehensive overview of your loved one's health. This information will be incredibly important during doctor's appointments, giving accurate and up-to-date data for better diagnosis and treatment decisions.

The "Keep Up with Your Loved One's Doctors All in One" log book provides a structured format to log your questions, concerns, and important information. It helps you stay organized and makes sure you don't miss any important discussions with the doctor. By actively participating in these conversations, you'll be better equipped to advocate for your loved one's needs and make informed decisions together.

I designed these books to help you get and stay organized, give you peace of mind, enhance the quality of care you provide and give you the confidence to navigate the healthcare system effectively. You can check them out on my website (along with vital signs equipment recommendations) at https://www.helpthecaregiver.com/store.

You should now be feeling confident about hospital follow-up appointments! Don't forget your copies of the MD appointment and vitals log books to help you stay organized.

Let's move on to the next important concern for new caregivers: Medications!

Now You Know:

- How to identify your loved one's PCP.

- How to research and find a PCP or specialist if your loved one doesn't already have one.

- Where to locate any appointments the hospital made for you on the discharge papers.

- How to reschedule any visits that need to be rescheduled.

- How to change a referral if you prefer a different doctor than the one initially referred.

- How to call any doctor's office you've been referred to in order to better understand the doctor's specialty and the reason for the referral.

- How to schedule a hospital follow-up appointment if it wasn't done by the hospital

- What you need to bring with you to these appointments

- How to make the most out of these appointments by preparing questions and logging vitals in advance

Checklist:

__ Identify your loved one's PCP

__ Locate any appointments that the hospital made for follow up after discharge

__ Call to reschedule any appointments that were made that need to be changed

__ Call new doctor's office(s) to clarify reason for referral, if you need to

__ Research and decide which new specialists you would like a referral for, if necessary

__ Make a note on appointment to-do list to ask for new referral(s) that are needed

__ Schedule any follow ups with specialists your loved one already sees that have not already been scheduled

__ Decide how you will track vital signs

__ Decide how you will organize MD and visit information

Notes:

#2 Organizing Medication

L et's break down how medications and hospitalizations are connected to help make sense of this section. Ideally, we'd never end up in the hospital. We'd have regular check-ups with our doctors, who would be aware of our health concerns. They would prescribe medications to address issues like high cholesterol, blood pressure, or blood sugar. If necessary, specialists would step in to manage specific conditions and prescribe additional medications related to their area of expertise.

In this perfect scenario, we'd take our medications as prescribed, and our doctors would follow up to make sure our symptoms were managed and our blood work stayed in a normal range. If anything changed, we'd report it to our doctors, who would make adjustments to our medication as needed.

All of your doctors would be informed about all of your care from your whole care team, and they would have a system of communication that would give a comprehensive overview of everything going on with you in one well-organized space. In theory, this approach would keep most of us out of the hospital unless we had an accident or planned surgery.

Sounds perfect, right? Unfortunately, reality often doesn't align with this ideal model for a few reasons. First, many people don't see a doctor until something is seriously wrong, often waiting way too long. Second, some people struggle with taking medications correctly, whether due to confusion about what to take, inability to afford their medication, or refusing to take medication for one reason or another.

Third, our bodies don't always give clear signals that something's wrong until it becomes an emergency. Fourth, while each medical facility has its own internal system for organizing patient information, different facilities typically have no way to automatically communicate with each other about your care.

Lastly, highly stressful events like the unexpected loss of a loved one or overwhelming new life circumstances can trigger medical conditions. This is something that can rarely be anticipated, but can have very big medical effects. Suddenly becoming tasked with full time caregiving (for example!) can create high levels of stress and anxiety, can drain financial and other resources, and can cause missed appointments of your own. Please make sure to keep your own health and well-being on your priority list!

All this to say, the reasons for hospitalizations aren't always clear-cut. Sometimes, we need to backtrack and do some detective work to figure out what happened.

Why Did My Loved One End Up in the Hospital?

Generally, one of three things occurred.

Scenario 1: Your loved one was taking all their medications as prescribed, yet they still ended up in the hospital. In these cases, there's likely been a change in their medical condition since their last doctor's appointment, and their medication needs changing. This is the easiest and most straight-forward case to address.

Let's explore the next two scenarios that can often create confusion and problems when it comes to changing a patient's medication list.

Scenario 2: The patient should have been taking their medications as prescribed, but they weren't. This could be due to various reasons like financial difficulties, uncertainty about how or when to take the medicine, or reluctance to take it due to unwanted side effects. Regardless of the reason, not taking the medications as prescribed led to a major issue where their body became severely imbalanced, resulting in hospitalization.

Scenario 3: The patient is being prescribed conflicting medications from multiple doctors. Due to incomplete or incorrect medication lists, these doctors are unaware of the conflicts and may unintentionally over-medicate or prescribe incompatible medications to the patient.

The lack of communication between different doctors' offices, as we discussed in the previous chapter, can be made worse by changes made at the hospital. This can potentially lead to recurring hospitalizations, because no one knows exactly what the patient is taking.

That's why it's so important for you to carefully go through this chapter and make absolutely sure you have an accurate and up-to-date master list of the medications your loved one is taking that can be shared with the primary doctor, specialists, and the hospital.

As we organize the medications, we want to better understand why the hospitalization occurred in the first place. This allows us to minimize the chances of it happening again and communicate effectively with the healthcare professionals involved in your loved one's care.

Throughout this process, things may seem more confusing before they become clear. You might come across old prescriptions, new prescriptions, generics, name brands, and varying instructions. Some medications may be temporary and others might be unclear as to which instructions are most up to date. Also, you might encounter situations where you need to stop taking certain medications and start new ones, but there are no instructions about what to do for future refills.

Hang in there! We're in this together and if you follow this chapter, you WILL get everything straightened out. I'll guide you through the process I use when admitting patients to home health, helping them figure out all these issues. **Follow along one step at a time, and we'll get you to the other side of this. I promise!**

This process can be straightforward if there are only a few medications involved or minimal changes, but it can also be as challenging as untangling Christmas lights! No matter which it is, we have to get clear about which medications the patient should and shouldn't be taking, and make sure that all doctors involved in their care have an accurate and up-to-date list.

When doctors consider prescribing medication, one of the most important factors they must take into account is the potential for conflict with other medications the patient is taking. If they are unaware of all the medications, they might unintentionally prescribe a medication that could have a negative reaction. It's not just about the heart doctor knowing the heart pills; they need to be aware of everything, including supplements and vitamins.

You should always have an updated master list of all the medications your loved one is taking. I highly recommend keeping a digital version that can be easily updated, as well as a paper copy that you can access easily. It's helpful to have copies in your wallet or purse, something you always carry with you, in case of emergencies.

Pro tip: Remember to include the date when the list was last updated. This way, if you come across multiple lists, you'll know which one is the most recent and accurate.

If you don't already have an organized list, you can access my FREE template that can be digitally edited and printed by going to https://www.helpthecaregiver.com/medication-list

Getting Everything Ready

Let's get organized!

Step 1: First, gather all the medications in the house. If your loved one has specific places where they keep certain medications, make a note of where you found each one to avoid chaos or potential arguments. Sticky notes can be very handy here.

Step 2: Get a piece of paper to take notes on and stay organized. If you'd like to use an organization chart I've created to help you with this, you can access it by downloading my FREE Medication Organization resource at https://www.helpthecaregiver.com/medication-organization

Note: We will address medications prescribed by the hospital and any changes recommended by hospital doctors, but only after completing the following process. We need a clean slate and a clear understanding of the pre-hospitalization medication situation before we tackle any changes related to the hospitalization.

Now that we have all the pre-hospital medications together in one place, we need to assess each one. If your loved one is like many of my patients, they may have outdated prescriptions or medications that are no longer part of their "active medication list," and they might not even remember where some of the prescriptions came from. Let's get to the bottom of each bottle, one at a time (deep breath! It's going to be ok!)

Finding Out What They Usually Take

Step 3: Ask your loved one how often they take each medication, one at a time. This step is important because you need to know how they are ACTUALLY taking the medication. The way they are supposed to take it, according to the label, may be different from how they are actually taking it.

Steps 3 & 4 - Organizing Existing Meds

Medication/ Supplement	Dose	How Often WERE they taking it?	How often were they SUPPOSED to be taking it?	What is it for? (What medical probelm?)	Prescribing doctor	Notes/Questions to ask the doctor	Add this medication to updated med list? (Yes/No)

From my "Organizing Medication" free download

Taking the extra time to go through these medications with your loved one will be incredibly helpful in the long run. Go through each bottle with your loved one and ask them how often they take the medicine and what it is for. Please be patient during this step, as they may need time to think or look at the pill to identify it. Many of my patients remember their medications by their appearance (size, color, and shape) rather than the names on the bottles.

If your loved one doesn't know how often they take a certain medication, move on to the next one. If they can't answer your questions about any of their medicine, or they are answering incorrectly, this is a safety issue. In this case, it's likely that someone else needs to be in charge of organizing the person's medications.

It's also important to note if they can only describe the medication based on its appearance. Pharmacies may change suppliers for a particular medication, resulting in it looking different. This change can cause anxiety or confusion for patients who rely on the way their pills look to stay orga-nized. If that happens, you may need to contact the pharmacy to confirm that it's the same medication and provide reassurance to your loved one.

As you go through the medications, pay attention to the prescription label. Note how often they are SUPPOSED to be taking each medication.

Step 4: Make a note about whether a) the patient is taking the med-ication correctly as prescribed/written on the label; b) they are taking the medication differently than prescribed/written on the label, and how they are taking it instead; c) refusing to take a medication they should be taking; d) this is an old prescription that no longer applies to the patient

If they are taking it correctly, you don't need to do anything else. You can mark this medication as ready to add to the updated medication list.

If they are taking the medication differently from what the label indicates, make a note of the difference between how they take it and the instructions according to the label. Most of the time, a patient is taking a certain medication less frequently than prescribed. It's less common for someone to take medication more often than they should, except for pain medicine.

Also, take note if they are **knowingly** taking the medications differently than prescribed. They might have a valid reason that requires further investigation. For example, they might be taking only half of their blood pressure pill to avoid dizziness or fainting.

If they have a reason for taking a medication differently than prescribed because they are experiencing bad side effects, write it down in the notes column and be sure to discuss it with the doctor. Remember, we're not trying to argue with your loved one right now, we just want to gather more information.

You may encounter medication that your loved one says they don't know about, or they don't know where they came from, or they don't take anymore. We'll address these shortly. **For now, set them aside** (we'll go through these next) and focus on dealing with the medicine they know they should be taking but are taking differently from what the label says.

If you need help understanding how to read a medication label or finding specific information on it, don't hesitate to ask the pharmacist to explain the labels on the prescriptions that are being filled at the pharmacy. You can also search online for resources on "how to read a medication label," or refer to the picture below to help you get started.

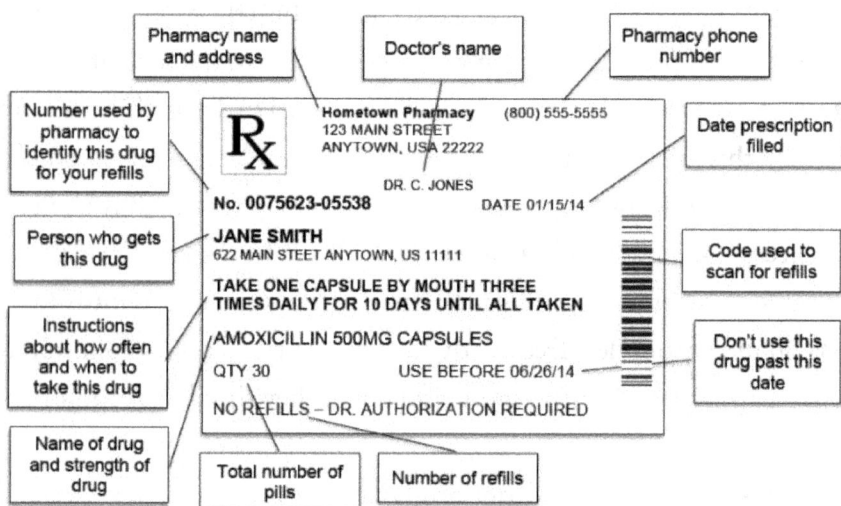

The different parts of a medication label

Communicating with the Doctor About Problems You Find

If you discover that your loved one is not taking a medication as often as prescribed, it's very important to make a note of it on your list. From here, you'll need to ask some additional questions, take notes, and potentially do some digging and call the doctor to figure out how to address this situation.

Always follow up with the prescribing doctor because they will need more information from you to make the safest decision for your loved one. Let's say your loved one has been taking their blood pressure medicine only once a day instead of the prescribed twice a day, but their blood pressure readings have consistently been in a healthy range. There's a possibility that taking the medication twice a day as originally prescribed might lower their blood pressure too much, which can also be a problem.

The same applies to medication intended to lower their blood sugar. Having very low blood sugar can become an emergency. If you simply call the doctor and ask how many times a day to take the medication, they will likely tell you to follow the instructions on the label. They need more information before making any further decisions, so make sure you are able to clearly tell them what's been going on.

Try to find out how long your loved one has been taking the medication differently from the prescribed instructions. For instance, if they have been taking only half the prescribed dose for six months and their blood pressure has remained healthy during that time, bring this up during the follow-up visit with the doctor.

Explain to the doctor, "When you first prescribed this medication, the prescription said to take it twice a day. However, Mom didn't realize that and has been taking it once a day. Whenever we check her blood pressure, it's always in a healthy range (show the blood pressure log). I'm concerned that her blood pressure might drop too low if she takes the medication twice a day. Should we continue with the current dosage or should we try taking it twice a day and keeping a log of blood pressure readings and report back?"

This example demonstrates how I want you to approach every medication problem you find. Changing a lot of pills on a person without keeping a close eye on things can create new problems. You need to rely on numbers. It may require some extra time and money to get new lab work done or monitor certain vital signs like blood pressure or blood sugar more closely, but it's still much less of a hassle than another hospitalization.

If it's a cholesterol pill that your mom has been taking once a day instead of twice, ask the doctor who initially prescribed the medication to order new lab tests to check her current cholesterol levels. It's the only way you be sure if she truly needs to take the second pill. Once you start her on the second dose, repeat the lab work as advised by the doctor.

Keep in mind that older individuals are generally more sensitive to medications, and most doctors are aware of this and prescribe accordingly. A certain dose of a medication prescribed to an 81-year-old can have a more significant effect than the same dosage given to a healthy person in their 30s. People with multiple medical conditions and lots of daily medications are more prone to experiencing negative side effects when their medications are changed.

It's much safer to find out current numbers (lab work, blood pressure, blood sugar, etc.), make changes or adjustments based on those findings, recheck after the medication has had enough time to take effect (which could be a few weeks or months later), and verify that everything is within a normal range. This approach is more reliable than making assumptions and changing things without knowing the numbers.

CHECKPOINT:

At this point:

- You have a clear understanding of all the medications your loved one was definitely taking before the hospitalization.

- You've made notes about any problems you found between how often they are taking a medication compared to how often the label says to take it.

- You have a plan for following up with the prescribing doctor(s) about any medications that need clarification.

Mystery Medication

Now, let's address the other bottles that you found, which your loved one says they either don't know what they are for, were told to stop taking, or don't know where they came from.

To make sure your loved one is taking exactly what medications they need to—no more and no less—we need to determine what to do with each of these "extra" bottles.

Step 5: For each bottle, make a note of: 1) who prescribed the medication, 2) the date it was filled, and 3) if there are any refills left. All this information is listed on the prescription label. From there, you can decide what to do with this medication.

Steps 5 & 6 - Mystery Medication

Medication/ Supplement	Dose	When was the prescription filled?	Are there any refills left?	What is it for? (What medical probelm?)	Prescribing doctor	Notes/Questions to ask the doctor (& which doctor to follow up with?)	Add this medication to updated med list? (Yes/No)

From my "Organizing Medication" free download

Sometimes, simply answering these three questions will provide the answer you need. You might recognize the doctor as a previous one your loved one no longer sees. In that case, you might realize that the medication is already on your list from the new doctor they are currently seeing. Mystery solved! The new doctor is overseeing that medication, and we don't need to follow up with anyone regarding the old bottle.

You might realize this is a duplicate of a medication that is already on your list, and all the information is actually the same. Now you know that these are the same, and you can organize them along with the current medication as extras.

You might discover that the prescription was filled several years ago. If you type the name of the medication into Google, you find out it's an antibiotic with no refills. Your loved one insists they aren't supposed to be taking it. It's not listed on any of the medication lists from the hospital paperwork or their doctors. It's likely that this medication is no longer relevant to your loved one's needs. It's always a good idea to double-check with the prescribing doctor, but in this case, it's likely not needed anymore.

If your loved one does not recognize the name of the doctor, ask if that might have been the name of a doctor at a hospital from a time when they were hospitalized. We will get to hospital doctors in just a bit. If you are not sure, see if you can type the doctor's name into Google, along with the city and state where you live or where the hospital is, and see what pops up.

If you STILL can't figure out who that doctor is, the next easiest thing to do is put that on the list of questions to ask the PCP at your follow up visit. Tell them, "We have (this medication) that was prescribed on (this date) by (this doctor). We cannot figure out who that doctor is and we are wondering if you were familiar with the name. Is this a doctor at the hospital? Or is it a specialist you might know of?"

If the PCP knows the doctor, he or she will gladly tell you. If they are not familiar, your next question needs to be about that medication and who should be managing it. Let the PCP help you figure out what to do next with regard to that medication. As I said, we will get to hospital doctors and medications in just a bit. Hang tight.

Hopefully, your PCP will be able to help you find out who the doctor is that has prescribed this medication, and if they are NOT a hospital doctor (often referred to as "a hospitalist") you can add them to your list of doctors that you need to follow up with, if needed.

Step 6: Gather all the bottles that need to be discarded in one place and mark them or create a system to recognize that you've already gone through them and confirmed they are not needed. Empty bottles can be thrown away or recycled. It's always best practice to remove the labels that have patient information on them first.

As for bottles with remaining medication, it's best to dispose of them at a "medication disposal/drug take-back" location. Many pharmacies offer this service. It's good to call ahead and confirm that your local pharmacy has this kind of program before making the trip to dispose of the medications, just to be sure.

The purpose of drug take-back locations is to make sure there is proper disposal of medicines, preventing them from entering the water supply or landfill and potentially harming the environment. It's especially important for addictive, toxic, or emergency medications to prevent accidentally effecting small children or others who could be seriously harmed.

By physically removing these medications from the house, you eliminate the worry of confusion or accidents related to taking the wrong medicine. You can feel confident knowing that you have reviewed all the medicines, understand their purpose and dosage instructions, and have taken necessary steps to prevent any accidents or bad side effects.

There is one exception to this rule, which involves medications that were changed at the hospital. We'll address this shortly, but first, let's do a quick check-in.

CHECKPOINT:

At this point:

- You know what to do with each of the "mystery bottle" you found.

- You have a plan to follow up with a doctor about any answers you still need about whether or not your loved one should be taking a medication you found.

- You have identified and removed all the old medicines your loved one should not be taking, creating a safer environment at home.

Now, this process may have revealed potential reasons related to medication that could explain why your loved one ended up in the hospital. It may have also generated a list of questions to ask different doctors during your follow-up visits.

Make sure your notes are thorough so you don't have to repeat this process, including what questions you need to ask the PCP and specialists at the post-hospitalization appointment(s). You can write these questions down in your "Keep Up with Your Loved One's Doctors All in One" log book ahead of the appointments to make sure you don't forget to ask!

Medication the Hospital Changed

Next, let's organize the medication changes that occurred while your loved one was in the hospital.

Step 7: Gather the discharge papers that were provided when your loved one came home from the hospital. In the previous chapter, you located these papers while reviewing the follow-up appointments.

Look for a section titled "home medications" or "home medication list" on the discharge papers. Each hospital formats this information differently, but it's common to find a list of medications with no changes in one area and a separate section or column indicating medications that have been changed, stopped, or added.

Take note of each medication that was changed, stopped, or added. We need to figure out the corresponding doctor you need to discuss each of these with. It is very important to understand that the doctors at the hospital are not going to be managing these medications after you are home. They are not going to be sending in for any refills, and they will not be doing any follow up interactions or lab work with your loved one after discharge.

Steps 7-9 - Hospital Changes to Medication

Medication/ Supplement the hospital changed	Changed? Stopped? Or Added?	Who originally prescribed this med?	Who will be ordering refills for this med?	Which doc do you need to follow up with about this?	Does that doc agree to these changes?	Add this change to updated med list? (Yes/No)

From my "Organizing Medication" free download

You need to make any medication changes that the hospital recommends, BUT you also need to verify with your regular doctors and specialists that they agree with those changes and have updated your medical records with their offices before you regard that change as permanent.

For this reason, I recommend that you do NOT get rid of any medication that the hospital told you to stop taking until AFTER

your follow up visit with the doctor who prescribed that medication in the first place. Set any medications you were told to stop taking to the side, clearly labeled not to take for now, but don't get rid of them until your regular doctor confirms to do so.

If your regular doctor instructs you to KEEP taking that medicine, you could have a terrible time getting insurance to pay for that medication again (if your normal refill isn't due for a while) and it could be a very expensive problem to fix.

So, it is extremely important that you follow up with every one of these changes with your regular doctors. They need to know about them, approve them, update them in their systems, and then make any further changes they think are necessary based on their knowledge and background of caring for your loved one.

This is another reason why scheduling your follow up visits SOON after coming home from the hospital is so important. You want a final verdict on any medication questions asap. Best practice is to schedule all these follow up visits within 2 weeks of discharge if at all possible.

Step 8: For STOPPED or CHANGED medication: Follow up with the doctor who originally prescribed these to you. For example, let's say the hospital told you to STOP taking Metroprolol (which is a blood pressure medication) and this medicine was prescribed to you by Dr. Patel, who is your Cardiologist. You need to follow up with Dr. Patel about the hospital's recommendation to STOP this medication.

In this example, Dr. Patel needs to be the final decision maker on which blood pressure medication(s) and doses you are taking. Show him/her the discharge packet from the hospital that will show all the changes that were made during the stay, and your vital signs log of daily blood pressure readings you have been taking, and let him/her give final instructions on what to do next about the blood pressure medication.

Step 9: For NEW medication: It is very important to understand that the hospital doctor will not be calling in any refills for new medications prescribed. You will need the PCP or specialist to continue these prescriptions if necessary, so you need to decide which doctor to follow up with about this new prescription.

If you're unsure which doctor or specialist to consult about a new medication because you aren't sure what the medication does, see if there is information on the discharge paperwork that explains the medication's purpose. If you can't find what you need on the discharge papers, try searching the medication's name on Google. You should find basic information about its purpose. Look for keywords like "heart" or "diabetes" to guide you in the right direction as to which doctor to approach for each medication.

If your search results say that this medication manages blood pressure, then the doctor that manages your loved one's blood pressure medication is the one to ask. The purpose here is to get a general understanding of which part of the body is being affected by the medication, but Google doesn't know your exact circumstances, and sometimes medication can be used for an "off label" purpose (one other than its original use), so don't take what you find as fact. Use it as a starting point.

You can always defer back to the PCP to answer questions about new medications that you are unsure about. They should be able to answer questions about what the medication is for, and who should be managing it. **Important: do not consider this step complete until you have confirmed which doctor will be managing that medication, and you have had a conversation with him or her about it. You need to know who to call when you have questions about that medication or need refills.**

You should have a follow up appointment scheduled with each doctor who will be overseeing any of these medication changes.

CHECKPOINT:

At this point:

- You are clear about which medicines were recommended to be changed, added, or stopped by the hospital doctors

- You have the name of the doctor who is going to be overseeing each one of these medication changes

- You have made notes to schedule an appointment with each of these doctors to discuss the hospitalization and what final instructions they have regarding these medication recommendations

Step 10: Once you are clear on the final list of medications your loved one should definitely be taking, at what dose, and how often, create a master list with all of this information. Be sure to put an "updated as of (date)" somewhere on the document. You can create your own, or use my free download by going to www.helpthecaregiver.com/medication-list.

Keeping Track of Medications

Once you have a finalized master list of the medications that are supposed to be taken, the next step is to establish a system for keeping track of actually taking them.

There are various methods you can choose from, but the key is to create a system that works for you. It doesn't matter which method you use as long as it makes sense to you and ensures that the right medications are taken at the right times.

Let me share a few popular options I've come across to give you some ideas. However, I don't consider any method better than another because everyone's brain organizes information differently. What works for one person may not work for someone else, so find what works best for you.

Method 1: A traditional "pill planner." These can be great for those who prefer to go through medications once a week, track things on a weekly basis (rather than daily), and set it up in advance. Pill planners come in a variety of options.

You can find color-coded pill planners for distinguishing between morning and evening pills, or ones labeled with the days of the week. They are available for once-a-day to four-times-a-day medication schedules, depending on your needs. Some have removable days, allowing you to take only the pills needed for a specific day when you have a doctor's appointment or will be away from home.

One drawback I've noticed with this method is for patients with memory issues. They may accidentally take pills from the wrong day because they can't remember the current day. Another issue could be individuals who can't resist constantly opening all the pill sections, either because they think they're helping, or because they can't remember what's already been done. This can cause stress and uncertainty about whether everything is in the correct order.

If the pill organizer works best for you but your loved one experiences these challenges, a possible solution is to hide the pill box and distribute the medications yourself. Alternatively, you can opt for a pill planner with removable days and provide them with only one day's pills at a time.

Method 2: Pill packs. Pill packs are highly convenient for many individuals, especially caregivers who find organizing medications overwhelming or patients with multiple medications to take throughout the day. Instead of individual bottles, the pharmacy delivers medications grouped by the time of day in a pack.

These packs are labeled based on the designated time, and their format can vary depending on the pharmacy. They can come as a large sheet (around 10" x 12") with the medication grouped in "bubbles" that you push to release the medication, or as plastic bags rolled up in a box, where you can easily tear out the next pack, similar to a paper towel roll.

The benefit is that you don't have to worry about organizing the medication because it comes pre-organized in the pill packs.

However, there are some drawbacks to consider:

Not all pharmacies offer this option, and switching pharmacies solely for this option can be stressful for patients who have a strong relationship with their current pharmacist.

Some patients may feel anxious about their medication not being in traditional pill bottles. They prefer the organized feel and being able to distinguish each pill individually.

If medication changes occur frequently, managing pill packs can become challenging as it's not as simple as replacing one bottle with another.

If you prefer a hassle-free and done-for-you approach to medication management, you can inquire about pill packs at your pharmacy. Contact them or visit the pharmacy and ask, "Is it possible to get (my loved one's) medication filled in pill packs or blister packs?" If they offer this service, inquire about the process. If not, ask for an explanation. Reasons could include their inability to provide this service, insurance coverage limitations, or other factors. Once you have the answer, you can decide on the next steps.

Method 3: Writing on the medication bottles. Some individuals, especially those with a small or medium number of medications, prefer to keep all their medicines in a box or structured basket, allowing easy movement between rooms.

They keep track of their medication by writing on the lid or label according to their preferred method. For example, they might write "AM," "PM," or "AM/PM" if they focus on when to take each medicine. Others may use "1x," "2x," or "3x" to indicate how often the medication should be taken.

The drawback of this method is that it becomes challenging to keep track once there are too many medications with various rules regarding timing. Another drawback is the potential to forget whether the medication was taken or not.

I've observed that individuals who prefer this method often have a set routine and tie taking their medication to another activity, such as eating breakfast or dinner, to help them avoid missing doses.

The grocery bag: I want to address this method because I know some of you may encounter it, and I hope to prevent any unnecessary conflicts. It may seem disorganized, haphazard, or like a disaster waiting to happen when you see someone keeping all their medications in a grocery bag or tote bag.

However, I urge you not to immediately dismiss this as an irresponsible way of managing medications. In my experience, when I ask individuals with a bag of pill bottles to explain how they take their medication, they are often able to provide more information than many of my other patients. They know what medications they are supposed to take, when to take them, and what they are for.

I'm not suggesting that this is the case for everyone, but don't assume that a bag of pill bottles is automatically a problem that needs to be changed. If your loved one follows this method, ask them to go through their medications with you. If they can accurately identify their medications, leave it as it is! Remember, the key is to have a system that WORKS. If it's not broken, don't fix it!

There are numerous other ways to organize medications, and you can also consider a combination of the methods mentioned earlier. Find something that makes sense to you and stick with it. If you realize that it's not working as well as you had hoped, keep making adjustments until you find a system that does work.

On that note, it's important to ensure that all of a patient's medications are filled at the same pharmacy. The pharmacist serves as a final safety net for identifying potential interactions. They should have a master list of all your active prescriptions, and if a medication is prescribed to you that has clear negative reactions with another medication, the pharmacist is supposed to double-check with the prescribing doctor to ensure they are aware of the potential interaction and still believe the prescription should be filled.

However, you cannot solely rely on this as a foolproof method. You need to be aware of medication allergies and be willing to ask the pharmacist questions about new medications. I often come across patients who are given prescriptions for pain medications to which they have a known allergy. Therefore, you must always be your own best advocate.

Use the Pharmacist as a Resource

Take advantage of your pharmacist as a valuable resource! Here are some great questions to ask your pharmacist about your medications:

Are there any of these medications that I should not take at the same time?

Should any of my medications be taken on an empty stomach or with meals?

Can you verify that this medication does not have any potential interactions with my current medications?

Does this medication contain any substances to which I'm allergic?

Are there any significant side effects associated with this medication that I should be aware of? Are there any red flag side effects that I need to report if they occur?

Is this medication safe for me considering my specific medical condition? It is especially important to double-check this if you have certain conditions such as being on blood thinners, having undergone a transplant, having cancer, or experiencing kidney failure.

Remember, the pharmacist does not take the place of asking these questions to the prescribing doctor, but they can provide additional clarification on any questions you may have not remembered to ask. They can also often contact the doctor more quickly than if you were to leave a message on a nurse line at the doctor's office.

Now, let's move on to home safety!

Now You Know:

- You now have a solid understanding of the medications your loved one should be taking and which doctor is managing each medication.

- You are prepared with any medication-related questions to discuss during follow-up appointments.

- You have a system in place for organizing and taking the medications that works for you and your loved one.

Checklist:

___ You have completed a thorough assessment of all the medications that were in the home prior to hospitalization

___ You know which prescriptions are current, and which bottles need to be disposed of

___ You have a list of doctors that need to be followed up with regarding medication questions, including questions about medication your loved one was taking incorrectly, medication they were refusing to take, and new/changed/stopped medication from the hospital

___ You have a list of specific questions to ask each doctor at your follow up visit about your loved one's medications

Notes:

#3 Home Safety

Alright, I understand that you're eager to dive into the logistics of bringing your loved one home from the hospital. However, I want to emphasize that I intentionally placed this section third on our list for a reason.

Things can quickly become chaotic once the process of bringing a loved one home from the hospital begins. You might become so focused on sorting out the things in this chapter that you forget to address the extremely important topics covered in the first two chapters.

If you felt the need to jump to this chapter first, I completely understand. However, I want to emphasize how important it is to go back and read the chapters about doctor follow-ups and medication management as soon as possible. These are time-sensitive issues that shouldn't be postponed any longer than necessary.

As we go through this chapter, I want you to create a list of the supplies you think you might need after going through each section. Write these things down in the "notes" section at the end of the chapter, or use the space on your printable digital copy of the Master Checklist at https://www.helpthecaregiver.com/home-from-the-hospital-checklist. The next chapter will focus on how to get the items you need, so don't worry: that information is coming!

I also want to remind you that the suggestions provided in this section are based on what has worked for many of my patients. However, it's important to note that this section does not substitute for a home evaluation by a physical therapist who can tailor recommendations to your specific situation. If you believe that you need a physical therapist to perform a safety and fall prevention evaluation for your home, please ask your doctor (almost all doctors can and will do this) to send a referral for a home health evaluation.

Basic Supplies

Let's move on to discussing basic equipment that you might want to consider having in your home. These items can be useful for everyone, but they are especially helpful when caring for someone with multiple medical issues.

Blood pressure cuff: This simple but important piece of equipment can provide vital information in emergencies or when your loved one experiences unexplained symptoms. One of the details that medical professionals will need to know in these situations is the person's blood pressure. Being able to track it immediately when symptoms start is extremely important.

Pulse oximeter: This device is essential for patients who use oxygen because it allows you to monitor their blood oxygen level at any given moment. Once again, if the person is experiencing concerning symptoms, this device can provide important information that you can give to a healthcare provider over the phone. These devices also measure heart rate, which is another important thing to monitor.

Thermometer: Being able to measure a person's temperature when they aren't feeling well is very important. Just make sure that you have a reliable thermometer on hand. Some are not as accurate, or are difficult to use.

Heart rate: this can be measured in several ways. An automatic blood pressure cuff will also measure heart rate. A pulse oximeter will display heart rate along with oxygen levels. Some smart watches can also be a reliable option! The most important thing is to make sure your device is measuring accurately, and use the SAME device every time.

Scale: If your loved one has a diagnosis of heart failure, takes lasix/water pills, or is having issues with losing weight despite eating, you might need to weight them regularly or daily to keep track of their medical status. Again, the most important factor is to use the SAME scale every time to increase accuracy.

Glucometer: If your loved one has issues with their blood sugar and/or they are diabetic, it's a good idea to have a glucose meter on hand to check their blood sugar at any time. This is especially important if they start having dizziness, become lethargic, or are difficult to wake up.

Medication organizer: After reading the previous section, you may have determined that using a medication organizer is the easiest way to keep track of all your loved one's medications. This can help ensure that the right medications are taken at the right times.

Gait belt: Also known as a "therapy belt," this is a canvas or plastic belt that is worn around a person's waist to assist family members or healthcare workers in safely moving the patient. It is recommended for patients who have a history of falls, experience unsteadiness while walking, or require assistance when getting up from a chair.

First aid supplies: It's a good idea to have basic first aid supplies readily available, including items like bandaids, gauze, wound cleaner, and disinfectants. Most pharmacies offer home first aid kits that you can purchase in-store or online.

Vital sign log book: As important as it is to have the necessary equipment to check your loved one's vital signs (such as blood pressure, heart rate, and oxygen levels), it's equally important to keep track of this information. Maintaining a log of these readings on a regular basis, even when your loved one is medically stable, can help establish a baseline and alert you to any potential changes that need to be reported to the appropriate doctor before an emergency occurs. You can create your own log, find printable templates online, or consider purchasing a logbook specifically designed for this purpose like the one I created, "Track Your Loved One's Vital Signs."

MD appointment communication book: With multiple doctors and various instructions to keep up with, it can become overwhelming to manage all the information. Many people resort to writing down notes on random scraps of paper or the backs of envelopes when communicating with healthcare providers. However, this can lead to disorganization and difficulties in finding important information when needed. Again, you can look online for an option you would like, or you can purchase the one I've specially designed, "Keep Up with Your Loved One's Doctors All in One."

If you would like to check out the log books I have created just for care-givers, along with all of my recommendations for the items listed above, you can find them on my website https://helpthecaregiver.com/store.

Please note that the above suggestions are not an exhaustive list, and your specific situation may require additional equipment. Now that we have covered the basic supplies needed for safety, let's discuss physical safety within your living space, including the ability to get in and out of the home, and moving around safely inside it.

Getting Into the House

When it comes to getting into the house, many individuals never consider the potential challenges until they or their loved ones are too weak to stand, walk, or climb stairs. Suddenly, it feels like an impossible task. If your loved one is unable to enter the house under their own power, even with assistance from family members, they may be brought home by EMS. While I appreciate the existence of this service, as a physical therapist and healthcare worker, it concerns me when patients find themselves in this situation at home.

The problem is that if they required EMS to bring them into the house due to their inability to do so themselves, they are at a high risk for injury or death if an emergency were to occur that required a quick exit from the home. Ensuring their ability to quickly exit the house becomes a top priority for me in these cases.

The solution may involve intensive physical therapy to help them regain their mobility, or it may require the installation of a temporary or permanent ramp. If their condition is expected to improve within a few weeks as they recover from surgery or a serious illness, it may not be necessary to install a ramp.

However, if their overall condition continues to decline or if they have experienced a stroke or other long-term injury that will require months of recovery, a ramp may be an important and necessary option.

Ramps are generally not covered by insurance, except for certain situations involving VA assistance. Therefore, if you require a ramp, you will need to explore ways to make it happen. Many times, local churches or charities will help build a ramp for an elderly senior in need. If your loved one is part of an organization like this, see if they might help build a ramp or donate materials. More information on potential resources for obtaining a ramp can be found in the resources chapter.

In this section, I want to highlight a few important qualities of ramps themselves. First and foremost, ramps can be wonderful but can also pose risks in certain situations. The biggest concern is having a ramp that is too steep. While I understand that properly installed ramps can require significant space, it is not worth compromising safety by having a ramp with a steep incline that puts the patient or anyone else at risk.

Whether the individual will be walking on the ramp or using a wheelchair, an angle that is too steep increases the risk of injury. It is important to adhere to recommended ramp installation specifications to ensure everyone's safety. If the patient is in a wheelchair and there is concern about the ramp, it is actually safer for them to go down the ramp backward.

Facing forward on a steep incline puts them at risk of toppling out of the chair, whereas slowly going down the ramp backward prevents this kind of accident.

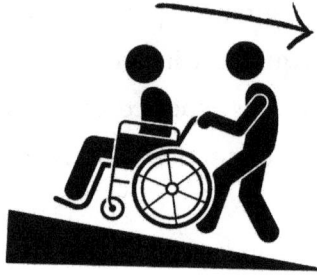

While ramps built to ADA guidelines should not have these issues, I have come across makeshift ramps where safety concerns were very real. For information on safe ramp building guidelines, see the resources chapter.

Adding grip strips or using old roofing shingles can be a cost-effective way to enhance the ramp's friction and prevent slipping, particularly in wet weather. Many patients have successfully used these solutions for added grip and safety.

Sleeping Arrangements

Sleeping arrangements can become overwhelming when there are no extra bedrooms available or if the only options require navigating a full flight of stairs. While each situation is unique and requires special consideration, I can share what I have seen work for my patients in similar situations where a bedroom on the ground floor is not available.

Safety should be a primary factor in making this decision. Consider whether the individual would be able to safely walk down a full flight of stairs in the event of an emergency if the only available sleeping arrangements are above the first floor. Some alternate options for sleeping include:

Converting a dining or office area on the ground floor into a makeshift bedroom. You can use curtains to create privacy in areas without doors.

Sleeping in a recliner or lift chair, which can be beneficial for individuals who have difficulty breathing when lying down or require assistance getting up. For information on insurance coverage for lift chairs, refer to the next chapter on obtaining medical supplies.

Utilizing a couch as a temporary solution if the person cannot safely navigate stairs and all the bedrooms are upstairs. While it may not be the most comfortable option, it can serve as a temporary fix until their strength improves.

Considering a hospital bed, which insurance will only pay for if it is medically justified or if you can afford to pay out of pocket. Hospital beds can be placed in a bedroom or an open living space such as a living room. For more information on getting a hospital bed, refer to the next chapter on Getting Equipment & Supplies.

In my experience with home health, I frequently help patients find solutions when their beds are not working for various reasons. Let's address some common issues and potential solutions:

Problem: The bed takes up too much relative space due to additional medical equipment, and there isn't enough space for caregivers to get around the room.

Solution: Push the bed against a wall, replace it with a twin bed or a hospital bed, switch bedrooms to a more accommodating space, or use a dining or living area as a bedroom until the patient becomes stronger or requires less medical equipment.

Problem: The bed is too tall, making it difficult or unsafe for the patient to get in and out of bed.

Solution 1: Check the bed frame to see if the mattress can be lowered. Some frames offer multiple height options that can be easily adjusted by someone capable of removing the mattress and using a screwdriver.

Solution 2: Remove the box springs, which can lower the bed by 6-8 inches. To provide support for the top mattress, add extra 1"x4" wooden slats or a plywood board.

Note: I do NOT recommend using a stool to get in and out of bed. For someone who is weak and/or medically compromised this is a huge fall risk. Please do not do this! Make me the bad guy here ("That physical therapist said no, mom!"). I can take it.

Problem: Furniture (e.g., chair, bed, couch) **is too low** for the person to easily or safely get up from, particularly for taller individuals.

Solution 1: If it's a chair, consider having a trusted friend or family member build a sturdy platform with a raised lip to prevent the chair from slipping off.

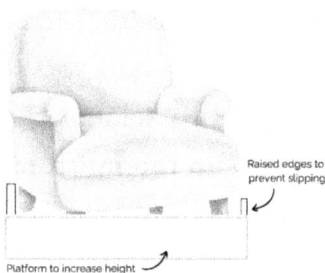

Raised edges to prevent slipping

Platform to increase height

Solution 2: For beds or couches, risers can be used to elevate the furniture legs. You can find examples of these risers on my website https://helpthecaregiver.com/store.

I have observed many patients who struggled to get out of bed due to prolonged use of one area of the mattress, resulting in a soft or sunken spot. Flipping or rotating the mattress can work wonders in terms of stability and making it easier to get into/out of bed, saving you the need to purchase a new mattress.

Bathroom Safety

Bathroom safety is so important, because it is one of the most common areas for falls in the home. Let's explore ways to minimize the risk of falls for your loved one in the bathroom.

Night lighting: Insufficient lighting at night can contribute to falls among the elderly because as we get older, our eyesight generally gets worse, which can lead to accidents. Make sure there is adequate night lighting in the bathroom and from the sleeping area to the bathroom at all times. Ideally, have lights that stay on or automatically turn on when it gets dark.

The toilet: Can your loved one safely stand up from the toilet? If not, consider using an elevated toilet seat, with or without handles for support. Another option, if you have a bedside commode, is to remove the bucket and place the seat over the toilet (lift the toilet seat to prevent mess).

The shower: Does your loved one need to sit down to shower safely? This is likely the case if they are weak and need help with bathing. Shower chairs and shower benches are available options. Benches are great for extending over a bathtub, allowing you to sit first, scoot your bottom back into the bathing area, and then bring your legs over the tub one at a time. However, benches require shower curtains to extend out around them, which can lead to water on the floor. Water on the floor definitely poses a fall risk, so plenty of towels will need to be used to keep the area dry and safe.

In some cases, there may not be enough space in the bathroom for a bench seat. This is often the case when the toilet is right next to the bathtub, on the end of the tub opposite the shower head. This set up creates an issue where the extra length of the bench cannot fit between the toilet and the tub.

Chairs can prevent water from getting all over the floor but require the ability to step over the sides of the tub, which can pose a fall risk if the person is unsteady. A walk-in shower with a shower chair is the best case scenario, if it's available.

Removable shower heads can be a fantastic investment for individuals who need to sit while bathing. The give control of the stream of water away from the person's face, and can help with better independence with bathing, because the person can aim the water toward their front, back, or hair in a way that is not possible with a fixed shower head.

Grab bars: These are great for supporting safe mobility in the bathroom but can cause trouble if installed incorrectly or if the wrong type is used. I do not recommend grab bars that "stick" to the wall with suction cups, even those with an additional button to increase suction strength. I have witnessed these bars falling off with minimal force, and I cannot comfortably recommend them as a safe option.

Permanent grab bars are the only ones I feel confident recommending. They may be slightly more expensive, but they are definitely more cost-effective than the consequences of a fall resulting in a broken bone. I would suggest investing in two super sturdy, well-placed permanent bars rather than having three or four cheap ones, with the risk of one falling off when your loved one really needs it.

I understand that the idea of drilling holes in the wall for installation is not always what you would prefer, but I have also witnessed patients falling into a wall so hard that it put a hole in the drywall. Holes made by screws are easier and cheaper to fix than holes caused by falls.

Grab bars should be installed in wall studs for maximum stability. Stud finders are available at hardware stores or online. If you have a knowledgeable friend or family member, they can also help you with locating the studs.

Determining where to place the grab bars depends on personal comfort and preference for your loved one. They are more likely to use a bar if it is installed in a way and location that feels natural and easy for them to use. During a home assessment, I often ask patients to show me how they currently get off the toilet and in and out of the shower. This helps me make recommendations that line up with their natural movements, avoiding the need to change their reaching, pulling, or pushing preferences.

When it comes to getting off the commode, different patients have different preferences and strategies. Some may grab onto a window sill, while others reach across to a counter or a shower door. Some patients push up from the handles on the elevated toilet seat and then try to turn towards their walker.

My goal is to facilitate their most comfortable and natural way of getting off the commode by adding a grab bar that lines up with the way they already prefer to move. For example, if they often try to grab a window sill to their right, I will suggest placing a grab bar beneath that windowsill. It allows them to perform the same motion using the same hand, but with the added support and safety of a bar to grip.

Similarly, if they attempt to reach for a shower door handle across from the toilet, I will look for a space on the wall beside the door where they can pull themselves up instead. Shower doors are not stable surfaces for supporting body weight and should not be pulled on.

When it comes to using the shower, if the person is using a shower bench, I'm not as concerned about grab bars. They should not find themselves in a standing position while in the shower or tub, so the risk of falling is minimized. It might be nice to have a handle in the bathtub for them to grab onto when rinsing shampoo out of their hair, but that is usually the only time many patients will need it.

However, if they are using a shower chair or insisting on standing, it is very important to consider grab bars for safe entry and exit from the shower area. I often have patients show me how they would normally get in and out of the shower, making sure to do this when everything is dry. This allows me to observe where they naturally reach for stability.

Are they trying to grab the edge of the shower before stepping in? Are they attempting to brace themselves against the far wall? It is important to support whatever method they feel is the most stable and safest for entering and exiting the shower. If they find themselves in an unstable position or feel like they are falling, they will instinctively use these familiar reaching and grabbing patterns, regardless of the placement of grab bars.

If they prefer reaching to the far side of the shower, is there a suitable location for a grab bar there? If they rely on gripping the edge of the shower, is there space in that area to install a grab bar?

For patients who are particularly weak or unsteady, it may be necessary to have two or even three grab bars strategically positioned to facilitate safe entry and exit from the shower. This could include a grab bar on the long wall of the shower or directly in front of them to assist with standing when they finish showering. Another grab bar might be needed on the wall just outside the shower, allowing them to hold on while turning into the bathroom to step out. A third grab bar at a distance from the shower could provide support while stepping onto the bathroom floor.

When it comes to getting in and out of the bathroom, many patients face difficulties due to specific circumstances. Some may need to use a walker, but the door frame is too narrow to walk through with a walker. Others may have a bathroom layout that doesn't allow space for a walker inside, which creates safety concerns if they cannot walk without one.

Some patients are capable of carrying a walker through the bathroom doorway by sidestepping through the door. As long as this method appears sturdy and safe, I do not try to change it. I'd rather have them use the walker than do without.

Some patients may not feel comfortable attempting to carry a walker through the narrow bathroom doorway and prefer to have a dedicated walker for their bathroom use. They keep this walker inside the bathroom and rely on their main walker to get through the rest of the house and up to the bathroom door. They transition from one walker to the other to stay stable and safe while inside the bathroom.

However, if the bathroom cannot accommodate a walker due to its narrow or small size, we explore the option of installing grab bars. Is there a need for a grab bar just inside the bathroom for them to hold onto once they let go of their walker? How do they navigate to the commode and shower area? By observing where they naturally try to grab for stability, we can determine strategic placements for grab bars in those areas.

It's important to note that the same grab bar can serve multiple purposes. You don't need a grab bar along every foot of the bathroom wall. Problem-solve based on the specific needs of getting off the commode, getting in and out of the shower, and getting in and out of the bathroom itself. Look for places where one grab bar can fulfill more than one of these needs. Remember, grab bars are a cost-effective measure compared to hospital visits. Fall prevention is the key priority here.

Stairs

When it comes to stairs in the house, they should only be used if it's safe to do so. While it may be inconvenient or uncomfortable to sleep in a different space from the typical bedroom arrangement, it's still better than being stuck in the hospital. Sometimes, sacrificing a little comfort now can prevent significant discomfort later. If stairs are a concern, your loved one may qualify for physical therapy to help them regain their prior level of function. Discuss outpatient or home health physical therapy options with their doctor.

If the patient can mostly handle stairs but has one significantly weaker leg, remember the therapy mantra for stairs: "up with the good and down with the bad!" The stronger leg leads when going up the stairs, and the weaker leg leads when going down. This approach makes sure that the stronger leg takes the brunt of the effort while descending, which is safer.

For more detailed instructions on safely going up and down stairs in this manner, including why descending with the weaker leg is preferable, go to my YouTube channel for a video demonstration.

If safety remains a concern, consider adding a handrail. Most stairs come with a handrail on one side, but it may be helpful to install a handrail on the opposite side as well. This provides a firm grip for the patient to hold onto with both hands. If your loved one is insistent about using the stairs despite concerns about safety, adding a handrail on the opposite side may be the best compromise to meet everyone's needs.

Oxygen

Oxygen plays a significant role in home safety because it poses both physical risks and requires certain precautions to avoid potentially serious consequences.

When it comes to compressors (the big machine that the oxygen is coming from), make sure they are positioned in a way that minimizes the risk of tripping. Make sure they are not in the middle of pathways where a person might have to walk around them, or where a walker or cane could accidentally get caught against them, increasing the risk of falls.

For oxygen tanks, there are several considerations to keep in mind. They should be stored upright, not lying on the ground. Either use a trolley specifically designed to hold them upright or secure the space where the tanks are kept in a way to prevent them from falling or being knocked over. This is especially important if there are small children or pets in the home who might accidentally tip them over.

Do not ignore or underestimate the risk of fire and explosion associated with oxygen use. Healthcare workers who have witnessed a patient after an oxygen tank explosion or fire stress the importance of taking proper precautions because they know how severe the consequences are. Avoid all forms of smoking, including cigarettes, vape devices, and marijuana, as they pose an immediate fire or explosion risk. Keep oxygen away from propane sources such as gas stoves, propane heaters, and grills. For more detailed precautions, refer to oxygen safety and information from lung.org provided in the resources chapter.

For the safety of visitors and emergency responders, consider placing a warning sign on your door indicating the presence of oxygen in the home. This alerts others to take appropriate precautions when entering, including refraining from smoking or using lighters.

Oxygen lines themselves pose a tripping hazard. As a physical therapist, it surprises me that people do not fall more frequently due to oxygen lines, but they do still trip and fall. I have encountered patients who have experienced serious injuries from tripping over oxygen lines, so let's discuss ways to minimize this risk.

Avoid using excessively long oxygen lines. Longer lines are more prone to tangling around your feet. Also, using an excessively long line can potentially result in less oxygen delivery through the nasal cannula or mask than what is being produced by the tank or concentrator. The oxygen concentration may decrease as it travels a longer distance between the concentrator and the person (for example, the tank is set on 3L of oxygen, but the person might only be receiving 2.5L by the time the oxygen reaches their nose).

Despite these risks, it is common for individuals to require extra feet of oxygen line to get around their space comfortably. I often recommend two solutions to patients: either move the oxygen concentrator to a more central location accessible from all the necessary areas (kitchen, bathroom, recliner chair, bedroom, etc.) or keep a shorter line on the concentrator most of the time and only add the extension line when they need to move throughout the day, such as when going to a bathroom located down a long hallway.

Apart from concentrator placement and line length, I frequently advise patients who require continuous oxygen to move a bit more slowly and carefully within their home. Taking extra time to look for the placement of the oxygen line, their walker or cane (if used), and their feet can make a significant difference in preventing accidents.

Floor Coverings

Floor coverings can create a fall risk, and managing them can be challenging for many patients and their families. I often find myself acting as a referee in between patients and family members when patients adamantly refuse to have their floor coverings picked up. Let me explain how I typically handle this issue.

The first concern with floor coverings is their movability. Mats or runners can easily slide or get tangled up with a patient's shoe, cane, or walker, leading to a fall. If a patient demonstrates any unsteadiness, scuffling when walking, or poor walker or cane management, I strongly insist that those floor coverings be picked up.

It surprises me how some patients absolutely refuse to pick up their rugs, even to the point of getting in major control battles with their families. If they are very unsafe when attempting to walk over these rugs or runners, but they are unwilling to pick it up, I make a compromise. I suggest using duct tape to secure the floor covering to the floor. It may not be the most attractive option, but I promise to let the issue go if they make sure the floor covering is duct-taped well enough to prevent any movement when they walk. For some patients, this solution is acceptable.

The other reason floor coverings can be hazardous is if patients fail to lift their feet, cane, or walker enough when walking over the edge of an area rug. The edge of the rug gets caught, and this sudden stop can cause stumbling or falls. If the rug is large and held down by heavy furniture like a bed, couch, or recliner chair, my concern is not about it slipping but rather about their ability to lift their feet properly.

If patients are successfully clearing the edge of the area rug without stumbling or tripping, I won't insist on removing it. In caregiving, we must choose our battles wisely, and area rugs are often not worth fighting over unless there have been instances of tripping.

During physical therapy sessions, I use this as a determining factor, giving patients a sense of control over the situation. I tell them that if they are effectively lifting their feet and are not stumbling or tripping over the rug edges, we will leave the rug in place and never mention it again. This motivates them to walk in a safer way and reduces the likelihood of conflicts with myself or family.

Getting Out of the House

Getting out of the house for doctor's appointments is another important aspect of home safety. We've already discussed entering the house and navigating stairs, but there may still be situations where the ability to leave the house for medical appointments is a major concern.

If the issue is having too many stairs and being unable to install a ramp, the main barrier may be safely navigating the stairs. In these cases, if you can get the patient safely into and out of a vehicle, you should be aware that emergency medical technicians (EMTs) can provide a "lift assist" specifically for doctor's appointments. This assistance involves physically helping the patient from inside the house to the driveway/vehicle and vice versa.

It's important to note that EMTs won't transport the patient to the appointment itself. That requires a separate resource that must be arranged several days ahead of time and is NOT free. For information about finding a ride to doctors appointments, go to https://www.patientsrising.org/how-to-find-patient-transportation-services/

Please note: in all areas I have worked in, lift assist services are free, but there are areas of the country where there is a charge for lift assist services, and it is important to be aware that charges for this service can change at any time. Please ask so you will know which is the case in your area.

If you need this kind of help, you can call 911 and let them know that you need a lift assist for a doctor's appointment, and the EMTs will be sent to help you. However, make sure to take into consideration extra time in your day for this.

If a patient is unable to get to a doctor's appointment independently, either because they don't have someone who can drive them or they can't physically get in and out of a vehicle due to weakness or a medical condition, you may need to arrange transportation to and from the appointment. For information about finding transportation to doctor's appointments, go to the link in the resources chapter.

Another option to consider is a telehealth visit. During the pandemic, telehealth visits became more common and started to be covered by insurance companies. This was a blessing that emerged from a difficult situation, allowing many patients to finally see appropriate doctors and specialists after years without access. With the status change of insurance covering this option, healthcare providers started offering telehealth visits more frequently. These visits count as regular visits and providers now have more flexibility to prescribe and treat through telehealth.

If your loved one has multiple appointments but lacks the time or stamina to attend them all in person, it's worth considering whether some of the visits can be made through telehealth. Contact the doctors' offices to ask about this option. If your loved one is physically too weak to leave the house and lacks transportation, tell the providers about these limitations. Some providers reserve telehealth visits for patients who cannot be seen in any other way, but it's always worth asking. Any visit is better than no visit.

If your loved one needs to be seen by a doctor or specialist, and telehealth is the only realistic option, but the current provider doesn't offer telehealth services, consider finding one who does. The key is making sure your loved one receives the care they need, and being seen through telehealth is better than not being seen at all.

Ok. We just covered so many great ways to make sure your love one is safe and has the supplies and equipment they might need. Make sure you have a list of all the items you need to get; in the next chapter, we will cover HOW to get the things that you need, so let's get started!

Now You Know:

- How to identify the medical and safety equipment your loved one needs for their care.

- How to complete a comprehensive safety assessment of the home where your loved one will be staying and how to troubleshoot potential safety issues.

- Alternate options related to getting your loved one to/from the doctor's appointments that they need to have for best care.

Checklist:

__ You have a list of any basic supplies you need to get

__ You know how your loved one will physically get into the house when they get home

__ You have a plan for making the entrance/exit from the home accessible (if needed)

__ You know which room your loved one will be sleeping in

__ You have a safety plan for sleeping (safe furniture height, safe furniture arrangement)

__ The bathroom is safe (to get into/out of the room, to get on/off the toilet, in/out of the shower)

__ You have a list of safety equipment needed for the bathroom (nightlight, grab bars, elevated toilet seat, etc)

__ You have a plan for stair safety (if needed)

__ You have a plan for oxygen safety (if needed)

__ You have a plan for floor covering safety (if needed)

__ You know how you will get your loved one out of the house for doctor's appointments OR you have an alternate plan (ex. telemedicine) to keep appointments until they are stronger

Notes:

#4 Getting Equipment & Supplies

N ow that you have a thorough and complete list of the equipment and supplies you will need, let's talk about how to get them all!

The first thing we need to consider is what insurance might cover. After all, if someone is paying for the benefit, it's important to take advantage of it! If your loved one does not have insurance, it's worth strongly considering helping them get it. If this is the case for you, you can find more information about getting insurance in the resources chapter. If there is no insurance in your situation, you can skip down to the section in this chapter about what to do for items that insurance doesn't cover.

Insurance

Before we dive into specific items, let me address a few notes on insurance. I understand that insurance can be overwhelming to understand and tricky to navigate. Even as a healthcare professional, I sometimes find myself confused and asking many questions.

However, I encourage you not to view insurance as the enemy. Instead, look at your loved one's insurance company as a partner in this journey. Approach them with the desire to learn more about how they can help while understanding their limitations.

It's important to remember that there needs to be a paper trail for every-thing, and any medical equipment or item must be justified by a doctor. Insurance won't simply deliver a hospital bed to everyone on your street just because they have coverage. There must be a genuine medical need for that item, and the doctor or specialist is the one to verify it.

Please note that not all insurances provide the same benefits or cover the same things. If your loved one has insurance through their employer, the company decided what the insurance package would look like for its employees. So, even if two people have the same insurance provider, their benefits may be different due to their employers' choices.

That being said, the insurance company still has many resources to support you, some of which you might not be aware of. **One of the best resources that many people do not know about is the option to have a personal case manager.** This person is assigned specifically to your loved one's case and they have medical knowledge to help navigate all of the different needs your loved one has.

Their job is to learn everything about your loved one's medical problems and needs, and be a guide through the process. Some insurances flag people with certain high-risk diagnoses, such as cancer, organ transplant, certain heart diseases, diabetes, etc, and assign a case manager automatically. But, regardless of your loved one's specific diagnosis, they can request that a personal case manager be assigned to them.

This dedicated person can help explain benefits, manage medical bills, provide education about medications, help with obtaining covered medical equipment, and much more!

If you're feeling overwhelmed by the amount of care your loved one needs and you're not sure where to start, don't hesitate to call the customer service number on the back of the insurance card and ask for a personal case manager to be assigned. You should be in contact with them very quickly, and they'll guide you through the process of navigating all these important matters.

And here's some more good news: you'll be given contact information for this person, so you can reach out to them directly without going through the regular customer service line. It saves you time and frustration – yay!

Working with a medical equipment company: if possible, try to get any medical equipment delivered through an in-network DME (durable medical equipment) company. While I hope this never happens, if an out-of-network medical equipment company delivers an item like a hospital bed or wheelchair, and the item doesn't work, (and the medical equipment company refuses to repair it), there might be nothing your insurance company can do.

However, if you use an in-network medical equipment company and encounter any issues, you can call the insurance company and explain the situation. They will help get it fixed for you. In-network providers have a contractual obligation with the insurance company to resolve any problems with the items they supply. Having the insurance company on your side gives you the power to get the issue resolved!

Now, how can you determine if a DME company is in-network? If you're tech-savvy, you can log in to your loved one's personal account on the insurance website and use the search tool to find in-network providers. Otherwise, you can call the customer service number on the back of the insurance card and ask for help with finding an in-network DME company in your area.

Sticking with an in-network DME company not only ensures support in case of any issues, but also helps you get the best price and maximum coverage, especially if there is a co-pay for the equipment or supplies covered by the insurance.

Now, let's discuss how you can find out what types of items could potentially be covered by your insurance policy. All insurance policies have publicly available "coverage policies." Your loved one's personalized coverage policy can be found by logging into their account or app with the insurance company and searching for it from there. This will be the most accurate document for your specific situation.

However, even if they don't have an online account, you can still view the insurance company's general coverage policy on their website by going to the site and typing "coverage policy" in the search bar. Keep in mind that this policy lists <u>potential</u> covered items, but coverage isn't guaranteed. For insurance to cover an item, there must be documented medical necessity, and the requirements for coverage will be listed on this policy document.

Warning: although I find reading these documents fascinating, they can be wordy and confusing for most people. I want you to know this document exists, but if you have questions about a specific item you think your loved one needs, and you want to know if it might qualify for insurance coverage, I encourage you to call the customer service number on the back of the insurance card and speak to someone about your questions. If your loved one has a personal case manager, feel free to contact them directly for assistance.

Items Ordered by the Hospital

If you have just brought a loved one home from the hospital, it's possible that you were told that the hospital would order certain medical equipment and send it directly to your house. This most often includes items like a hospital bed, wheelchair, walker, or bedside commode.

While most of the time, items ordered by the hospital are taken care of without any problems, there are a few issues that can come up, which I often see in my work in home health. It's helpful to keep in mind that there are three key players involved in getting medical equipment through insurance: the insurance company, the doctor writing the order for the equipment needed, and the DME company responsible for delivery (and possibly servicing the equipment).

For the order to go through successfully, a doctor must write the equipment order, usually with supporting documentation stating or showing that the requested equipment is medically necessary. If the doctor does not write the order, or if the order is incomplete, or if the supporting documentation is not sent in, or if your loved one does not meet the coverage requirements, the order will not go through, and you will not receive the equipment you were expecting.

Even if the doctor's order is correct, if the requested item is not covered by your insurance policy, the insurance company will deny the request. For example, if the doctor writes an order stating that it is medically necessary for you to have a Jacuzzi delivered to your house, but your insurance does not cover the cost of Jacuzzis, unfortunately, you won't be getting a Jacuzzi. Sorry!

Also, if a DME company does not receive the sent order (for instance, due to a fax not going through), they will not be aware of the request, and it could fall through the cracks. If the company is out of the requested item or doesn't carry it, the order might not be fulfilled for various reasons, including someone putting the request on a to-do list for follow-up that never gets done.

If your loved one has been home for several days and the item still has not shown up, and you haven't heard anything from anyone about it, don't hesitate to reach out to the DME company to follow up on the status of the order. If the hospital sent an order for these items to be delivered, they should have provided contact information for the DME company so that you would know who to call with questions.

If the DME contact information has been lost, and you aren't sure which company is supposed to be taking care of the order, you can call the hospital and ask for this information. You will need to be able to provide the room number the patient was staying in, or at least which floor or part of the hospital they were in when they were discharged, so that you can be sent to the right person who will have access to their chart. They can look at the notes and see which company the order was sent to.

The people at the insurance company will have the best information about any potential problems with approving an order, so reach out to them first with questions related to whether or not a piece of equipment can be or has been approved for coverage. If a request has been denied, the insurance company needs to be contacted to find out why and if there is anything that can be done to appeal the denial (maybe the paperwork was incomplete, etc).

The DME company is the main source for questions about equipment cost (rental versus purchase), how long you have to change your mind about wanting a piece of equipment, what to do if an item breaks or is defective, etc. Specific questions about the equipment features need to be directed to the DME company. The insurance company is only giving a yes or no on coverage. The DME company knows the details of the equipment inside and out.

After the order is sent, the doctor's office should only be contacted if the insurance or DME company needs something else from the doctor. They might need a copy of the most recent office notes, or a statement from the doctor confirming that an item is medically necessary, or maybe confirmation of the patient's height or weight at their last visit if they need specialty items related to these things, etc.

Insurance policies change frequently, and doctors are not able to stay up to date on every single policy and requirement change of every insurance policy in existence. It's just too much for them to dedicate their time to because there are so many variations and frequent changes. Every doctor's office I've ever called about equipment for a patient has basically included a question similar to, "so what exactly does this order need to say? Is there any other information that needs to be sent with it?" They are very willing to help, but they can't read the insurance companies' minds.

If the insurance company denies something because they need extra information from the doctor, be kind and patient when calling the doctor's office. They're not leaving out the information on purpose. They want the patient to have what they need!

Here are a few last "fun facts" about insurance coverage and equipment to help you understand the limits you might be up against, and how to make the best decisions when it comes to getting the equipment your loved one needs:

It can be challenging to understand exactly what insurance will cover, and what you can confidently purchase without waiting for insurance involvement. Keep in mind that insurance won't pay for items because they're convenient. For example, they won't cover two walkers just so you can keep one in your car. While it might be convenient, it's not medically necessary. They will expect you to buy the second one if it means that much to you.

Insurance also sets limits on how often they'll pay for certain items. For instance, many insurance companies will only cover one walker every five years. If they've already paid for a walker from a surgery you had two years ago, they'll assume it's in good condition and that you still have it, and won't cover a new one if you need it this year due to an accident.

I always advise my patients to hold onto the big equipment covered by insurance. Keep it in a back room, a closet, or find a way to store it. You don't want to be in a position where you need it again in a few years and don't qualify for another one.

Hospital beds and wheelchairs typically have a waiting period of five years before you can qualify for another one covered by insurance. The exception is if there's a significant change in your physical status or medical condition that requires a different type of bed or chair to accommodate increased need for support, or advanced features.

Some items can be sent immediately (meaning deliver it now, figure out the insurance later), while others require pre-authorization from the insurance company before delivery. A pre-authorization means the insurance has to be contacted and give an official "yes" on a request before the item can be delivered. Hospital beds and wheelchairs are often on this list and policies may vary between different companies.

If you want to know if an item could potentially be covered by your insurance and what information the insurance company would need for approval, contact their customer service. You can do this by calling the number on the back of the card or using digital communication methods like a chat feature on their website or a phone app.

Major items that are typically covered (if they are medically necessary), include hospital beds, wheelchairs, walkers, bedside commodes, and after-surgery braces.

More Insurance Rules

- Insurance won't cover a Rollator walker (the one with 4 wheels and a seat) but will cover a regular walker with two or four wheels. They won't cover accessories for the walker, like a tray or cup holder.

- Insurance won't pay for both a wheelchair and a walker. The idea is that medically, you should only need one or the other. If you really feel that you need both, have insurance cover the wheelchair, because they are much more expensive.

- For a bedside commode, documentation is needed to show that the patient is unable to safely reach the bathroom. And, insurance usually will only cover a "3-in-1" commode, which can be used as a bedside commode, a shower seat and toilet seat lifter, and features a removable bowl under the seat lid.

- Wheelchair coverage requires seat and height measurements, and for non-standard sizes, documentation is needed for height or weight over 300 pounds, in order to get approval for a narrow or wide chair.

- If bariatric equipment is needed, the order must specifically state "bariatric" for insurance to cover it.

- Walker leg extensions are available for individuals over 6 feet tall, but the height must be documented and specifically requested.

- To qualify for a hospital bed or wheelchair, the patient must be physically seen by the doctor writing the order. Because of this, it's best if the hospital doctor orders these items before the person goes home after an accident or major illness.

- Once the patient has been discharged from the hospital, they are no longer under the care of the doctors there, and it is very difficult or nearly impossible to get these items ordered from those doctors after the fact. So, if you originally told the hospital, "no, we don't need a wheelchair," and then get home and realize you actually do need it, the patient's PCP is the person to ask about the order.

What if the Item Delivered is Not the Right One?

Once an item is delivered to you, any issues should be addressed directly with the DME (durable medical equipment) company. They should be your first point of contact for all questions and concerns.

When an item is brought to your home, there should be accompanying paperwork that explains the terms and conditions related to the delivery. I highly encourage you to read this contract carefully and ask for clarification on anything you don't understand before signing for any equipment.

If you notice right away that the item being delivered is not the right one, do not sign for or accept the delivery. Signing for something makes it harder to correct any mistakes or misunderstandings later on.

The DME company will deliver whatever the doctor ordered. If the doctor's order was incorrect or missing important information, such as the need for the item to be a bariatric version, the DME company wouldn't know this, and they cannot legally alter the doctor's order. In these cases, a new and corrected order would have to be written.

Similarly, the DME company is bound by what your insurance will cover, unless you are willing to pay out-of-pocket and waive insurance involvement altogether. If the doctor orders something, but the insurance denies the request, the DME company cannot override the insurance decision.

For example, let's say the doctor ordered a bariatric walker, but the insurance denied it because the required weight documentation wasn't provided. Because of this, the DME company may attempt to deliver a regular-sized walker, which is what the insurance approved, but not what the patient needs.

If you receive the wrong item, don't panic. We just need to ask a few questions. First, check if it was a simple oversight by the DME company. Can they verify the type of equipment the doctor ordered? Can they confirm whether the insurance approved the item you were expecting?

Depending on the answers to these questions, you might need to call the doctor's office and request that an updated order with the necessary information be submitted to the insurance company. If the doctor's order is correct, but the insurance denied the request, call the customer service number on your insurance card and speak to a representative. Explain the situation and ask about the insurance denial and the reasons behind it. If you need to, you can start the appeal process to request that the insurance company reconsider, or you can provide them with more information that might change their decision.

The insurance company might explain that they don't cover the exact item ordered and provide reasons for the denial. Or, they may tell you that they can cover the item, but certain documentation needs to be submitted by the doctor first. If that's the case, you should call the doctor's office, let them know about the insurance denial, and request the necessary information to be sent.

For those with home health services, please understand that the home health company acts as a middleman in these situations. Although the home health company may make recommendations to the doctor's office, they are not the ones ordering or delivering the equipment. The doctor still has to write the order and send it to the DME company for insurance approval.

If you accept a delivery and later realize the item is incorrect, this can be a significant problem. If you are only renting the item from the DME company, it will be easier to fix. However, if the item was a one-time purchase covered by your insurance, and you now own the equipment, your options might be limited. It's worth contacting the DME company to explain the situation and ask if there is anything that can be done. Keep in mind that once you've signed the paperwork and accepted the delivery, your options may be limited.

Braces

I often get asked about insurance coverage for braces. If you have had surgery or a recent injury that requires a brace as part of the recovery process or for protection and safety, insurance will almost always cover these items, and you'll likely receive them before leaving the hospital or orthopedic doctor's office.

However, if the brace is not immediately necessary for post-surgery recovery, the process of getting it covered by insurance can be more complicated. As with all insurance-covered items, the doctor needs to write an order for the brace, justify its need, and send it all to the insurance company. The insurance company has to approve it, and a DME company will need to be involved in delivering it to you.

If your loved one has an insurance benefit similar to the over-the-counter benefit mentioned above, there may be some braces in that catalog that the insurance will cover without a prescription, such as a soft support brace for knee pain.

However, you can find many braces online for around $30, and I often encourage my patients to purchase them this way due to the low cost and quick delivery. However, if money is tight, or the item is higher in price, going through the doctor and insurance may be worth considering. You can find my recommended knee brace for patients with knee pain and those who complain about falling due to their knee "giving out," on my website at www.helpthecaregiver.com/store.

Lift Chairs

There can be a little bit of misunderstanding when it comes to insurance and lift chairs, so I want to touch on that quickly. Many insurances have some benefit related to lift chairs for those who need one because they are too weak to stand up out of a regular chair, and need the assistance for medical reasons. However, insurance does not pay for the chair itself. What they cover is a certain dollar amount that technically is going toward the motor in the lift chair. I know that may sound crazy, but the chair itself is not considered medically necessary, it's the motor that allows the chair to lift the person up safely that is considered a covered medical expense.

The way this works is that you 1) call the insurance company to learn what the exact benefit amount is and if there are any specific companies you have to order the chair through (like La-Z-Boy), 2) go to the furniture store and explain that you want to purchase a chair that is eligible for the insurance benefit (they will probably need some insurance information), 3) purchase the chair out of pocket, and then 4) file a claim for reimbursement for the amount of the benefit by going online to start the claim or calling the customer service line and starting the claim over the phone.

Each insurance policy may be different on how much money they will cover toward the cost of a chair and how the process works to get the chair covered. Call them first, call them to clarify during the process if you need to, and call them when you are ready to file your claim. You will still come out of pocket on most of the cost of the chair, but getting several hundred dollars back in your pocket is worth the time to take advantage of this benefit, if your loved one has it.

Insurance allowance

If your loved one has Medicare, a Medicare alternative, or Medicaid insurance, they likely have an "over-the-counter" quarterly allowance. They should have access to a physical or digital catalog listing all eligible items that can be ordered using this allowance.

For more information on this benefit, including how the program works, the amount available to spend quarterly, and how to access the catalog, you can call the customer service number on the back of their insurance card or log into the online account and search using the term "allowance."

Typically, there's a wide range of items to choose from, such as diabetic support items, stool softeners, eyedrops, first aid supplies, and more. Every little bit helps, so take advantage of this benefit!

What if There is No Insurance, or Insurance Doesn't Cover Something That is Needed?

The quick and easy answer is to visit a local pharmacy or browse online for the items you need. Most local and chain pharmacies carry commonly needed medical equipment on their shelves. Items like an elevated toilet seat, walker, Rollator with a seat, bedside commode, cane, etc., are readily available at these pharmacies.

Feel free to pick your favorite brand or find well-reviewed options. If you want my recommendations to reduce the amount of research you need to do, you can find them on my website www.helpthecaregiver.com/store.

If you're wanting to reduce expenses, especially for items you only expect to need for a short period, I often recommend that patients look at local second hand stores like Goodwill. They frequently have walkers, wheelchairs, and canes available because people often donate items they no longer need.

In some areas, Goodwill even has a rental program to provide medical equipment to those in need. It's worth calling around to your local secondhand shops to see if they have what you're looking for.

Another great option is to explore garage sales and estate sales. However, be careful not to pay high prices. Sometimes I've been shocked to see the asking price on used equipment that isn't in great condition, but you can also find great deals on equipment by visiting these sales.

I personally like to pick up wheelchairs, bedside commodes, elevated toilet seats, and walkers that I find at local sales. I keep them and give them to some of my patients who have the highest level of financial need.

If the patient needs a lot of equipment, but is expected to only need these items for a short time, consider asking around if someone has an item that can be borrowed. I'll be a little hypocritical here though, and encourage you to be cautious when lending out your own medical equipment.

Remember that insurance typically covers these items only once every five years, so only lend out something you can afford to potentially lose. I've had too many patients who were wanting to do a kind thing by lending out a piece of medical equipment, only to never see it again.

If insurance will not pay for a hospital bed, but you feel that your loved one needs one, you can look into second hand options, see if you know someone who will lend a bed they are not using, or consider using an option such as a Care Credit card to pay for one out of pocket. Keep in mind that if your loved one qualifies for hospice, they will cover the cost of a hospital bed.

If money is a barrier to getting needed supplies, check out the resources chapter at the end of the book.

Items that Insurance May Not Cover

If your loved one has an over-the-counter benefit, as mentioned above, you might be able to get certain items that your insurance will pay for and send to you with your quarterly allowance. You can get a lot of great essentials that way, so it's worth checking there first. Otherwise, insurance **generally will not cover** any of the following items:

- First aid supplies

- Vital signs equipment

- Therapy belts, therapy bands, or other physical therapy or occupational therapy equipment

- Bed pads, diapers, or most other personal care items

If your loved one has certain diagnoses, there may be exceptions to the above list. It's always worth calling the customer service number on the back of the insurance card to ask if there are specific items that your loved one qualifies for based on their diagnosis. For instance, glucose monitors or supplies for someone with diabetes, diabetic shoes, a scale for daily weighing for someone with heart failure, etc.

Again, if you would like my recommendations related to any of the items that insurance does not cover, you can find them on my website at www.helpthecaregiver.com/store. For other resources that can help cover the cost of these items for those with financial hardship, see the resources chapter at the back of the book.

Hospice Coverage of Medical Supplies

If your loved one is a potential candidate for hospice, I would highly encourage you to speak to a hospice professional about your loved one's situation and medical supply or equipment needs.

Hospice covers a wide range of medical equipment and supplies that are not covered under any other resource or insurance. Hospice will cover the cost of medication, a hospital bed, diapers, bed pads, etc. Speaking to a hospice representative can help to clarify all of the benefits available through hospice, along with addressing your questions and concerns.

There is never any obligation to transition to hospice just because you have spoken to a hospice representative about your options. Hospice can be an amazing blessing for so many people, and I have highly encouraged many of my patients who were appropriate candidates to consider and transition to hospice services.

If you would like to speak to someone about your options for hospice, you can let the primary care doctor know, and they can arrange to send someone out to speak with you. You can also research and contact hospice companies directly. They will send someone to your house quickly to answer your questions, without obligation to sign on to their services.

If the policies of that company are not in line with your/your loved one's needs or preferences, call a different company and explain your concerns. Ask if they have the same or a different policy than the one that you didn't like. Don't settle for an answer that doesn't feel right. There are many wonderful hospice companies out there whose team are absolute angels. Keep going until you find one that is a good fit. You won't regret it.

Now You Know:

- How to follow up on items ordered by the hospital

- What to do if an item that is delivered is not the right one

- Basic rules about what insurance will and won't cover

- Basic requirements for how to get something approved through insurance

- How to get items that are not covered by insurance

- That hospice can be an amazing option to help cover the cost of medical equipment and supplies, if your loved one is a candidate

Checklist:

__ You have located the patient's insurance card and the customer service number on the back of it

__ You have requested a "personal case manager" through the insurance and let them know about the patient's needs, including medical equipment and supplies (if applicable)

__ You know the name of the DME company that is being used for equipment and their contact number

__ You know what equipment has already been ordered and when it should be arriving

__ All the major equipment needs are ordered or have arrived (hospital bed? wheelchair? walker? bedside commode? oxygen equipment?)

__ You have checked for any quarterly allowance benefit the patient might get, and used it to order needed items

__ You have a list of items insurance doesn't cover, but that your loved one needs for safety or convenience (any of the major items that are not "medically necessary," a rollator walker with a seat, grab bars, night lights, personal care items, etc)

__ You know how you are planning to get the items insurance doesn't cover

Notes:

#5 Staying OUT of the Hospital

Your loved one has been through so much, and so have you! The last thing anyone wants is for your loved one to end up back in the hospital. This is exhausting, scary, expensive, and incredibly stressful.

In this section, we are going to go over the top reasons a person might have to return to the hospital after coming home and what to do to prevent that from happening. If you've made it to this point in the book, you are a million miles ahead in the game!

You know how to follow up with all of the appropriate doctors. You know how to use your pharmacist as a resource. You have all of your loved one's medication well organized, and all questions about the medications organized and ready to communicate to their doctors.

You know that the home living situation is safe, and there is an action plan for anything that needs to be done to increase the safety in the home. You also know how to use the insurance and/or community resources and online shopping to get anything for them that they need for their medical care.

Look at you! You are doing an amazing job!

Now, I'm going to give you the information you need to help manage the medical conditions that they might have that can cause them to become unstable and have to be readmitted to the hospital. The next two chapters cover dizziness and falls. If you have questions or concerns about those two things, they are coming next!

Your loved one will not have every issue on this list. They may only have one or two, or they might have other medical conditions that you are concerned about. This section is meant to address the issues that are most likely to cause a person to end up back in the hospital.

I can't possibly cover everything I would love to tell you in one book, but if you have questions or concerns about other conditions not listed in this chapter, please join my free Facebook group for caregivers: facebook .com/groups/caregiversofaginglovedones. You can ask your questions and share your concerns there. You might also find an answer to your question on my YouTube channel: youtube.com/@helpthecaregiver.

Here are the topics addressed in this chapter:
- CABG (heart bypass surgery)
- CHF (heart failure)
- Heart attack
- COPD
- Pneumonia
- Total hip or knee replacement
- Back surgery
- Preventing infection after surgery
- Blood clots
- Pain medication
- UTIs

Anytime there is a surgical wound, there is potential for infection. Please refer to the section in this chapter about preventing surgical infections for more information.

Anyone who has had surgery is at an increased risk for a blood clot. Please refer to the section about blood clots for more information.

After surgery, it is common for someone to be prescribed medication for pain. Please see the section about pain medication for further information.

One last note: the items being brought up in this chapter are assuming that this was the reason the person was originally put in the hospital, or it is a condition that regularly gives them problems and could contribute to them needing to go back to the hospital. If this is a condition or surgery that they had decades ago, and it doesn't give them any problems now, then the information in that section is less relevant for them at this time.

Having worked in home health for many years, I also know the contributing factors that can cause a lot of problems and complications for these conditions that may not otherwise be known by other healthcare professionals. If something I bring up seems unlikely, I promise you it is something I have seen with my own eyes more than once in someone's home.

CABG – "Heart Bypass Surgery"

CABG - The patient had "heart bypass" surgery. These letters stand for "Coronary Artery Bypass Graft" and is necessary when someone has a heart blockage (coronary = heart). If one of the arteries that carries blood to the heart is mostly or completely blocked, they will need this surgery to prevent them from having a major and very damaging heart attack.

To put the surgery in plain language, the artery is so bad that it can't be fixed, so the surgeon has to reroute the blood flow, kind of like the way police officers will redirect traffic around a bad wreck, and that rerouting is called a bypass.

In order to create this bypass, the surgeon has to use a blood vessel from somewhere else on the patient's body. It could come from the leg, chest, arm, or belly. This is referred to as the "donor site," and the patient will have a surgical cut in this area too.

In order to do the surgery, the surgeon has to cut through the sternum to get access to the patient's heart. As a physical therapist, one of my jobs is to make sure the patient understands the precautions they need to take when it comes to movement after this surgery.

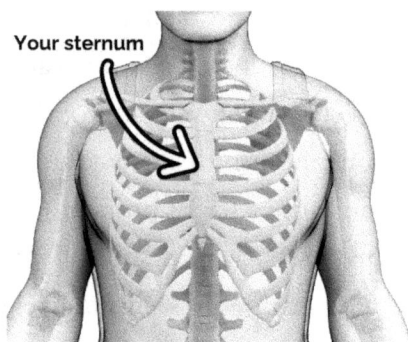

Your sternum

The sternum is typically a very strong bone, but it has been cut in half from the surgery, and needs a lot of time and rest to heal. The surgeon will sew the two halves of the sternum back together, but the bone is very weak after surgery, and this is something that needs to be taken very seriously during the healing process.

If there is too much stress placed on this freshly cut bone, there is a good chance that the surgical stitching will not hold, and the wound can burst open. If this happens, the person has to immediately go back to the hospital and will likely end up with a wound VAC in their chest, because the wound is so open that it can no longer be stitched back together. This is very serious and pretty scary, and I've seen it happen to a handful of patients who were not careful about their precautions.

What are the precautions? I like to answer this question by first explaining WHY the precautions are there. It is not possible to move your shoulder without also moving the muscles in your chest. Go ahead, I know you're trying it!

It's also not possible to push through your arms or pick up something that's heavy without activating the muscles in your chest. Feel free to try that one too! Put one hand on your chest muscle and push through your other hand. Do you feel the muscle in your chest activate?

Those muscles in your chest attach to your sternum. If the muscle is being activated, it is pulling on the sternum. If too much pressure is put on this newly stitched-up sternum, the stitches will pop. You don't want to overstretch the muscles for this same reason.

This is why it is extremely important that the person not push with their arms at all when they need to stand up out of a chair. They absolutely have to use their leg strength only to stand. Working with older and weak patients the way that I do, I know that this is often easier said than done, but it is just as important no matter how weak or sick the patient is.

If the person is weak, do not under any circumstances pull on their arms to try to help them stand up. Use a gait belt (which I commonly refer to as a therapy belt) to fit very snugly around their waist and help to pull them up from the belt. If the person is on the larger side and one therapy belt will not safely secure them, you can purchase an extra-long gait belt, or you can hook two of them together.

Many hospitals will send patients home with this kind of belt after this surgery, but if yours didn't, you can easily find this belt online. They are very inexpensive, and you can see an example of one on my website.

Your loved one should have been given a list of sternal precautions by their surgeon, but if they did not receive one, here is the list of standard precautions. As with anything, please double-check with the surgeon about your loved one's precautions or any post-surgery instructions.

Standard Precautions:

- No pulling or pushing through the arms

- No raising the arms higher than 90 degrees (because it stretches the muscle too much)

- No lifting (the weight limit can vary depending on the surgeon and any surgical complications, but 5 lbs is a safe assumption; check with the surgeon!)

- No reaching the arm behind the body (again, it's too much stretch)

- Support the incision with a pillow when coughing and try to reduce the force of the cough

How long are they on these precautions? Generally, these precautions are in place for 6 to 8 weeks after surgery, but you absolutely must ask the surgeon to clarify the timeline for your loved one, specifically. If the surgeon has not already said how long to mind these precautions, ask at the surgical follow-up visit, which should be before or during that 6 to 8 week timeframe, or call their office and leave a message for the nurse asking how long to expect the restrictions to last.

What else do you need to know to maximize recovery after this surgery?

- Having diabetes or smoking cigarettes will delay the body's ability to heal. If either of these things applies to your loved one, it's important to understand that they may need to be cautious with their sternal precautions a little bit longer.

- Make sure to take blood thinners and Lasix (water pills) as prescribed after this surgery to avoid very serious complications.

- Use compression stockings and keep the legs elevated frequently to help manage swelling in the legs after this surgery. Having too much fluid in the body can put strain on the heart. The heart just went through a lot with this surgery and will not handle extra demand very well.

CHF -"Heart Failure"

CHF - The patient has "heart failure." Here's the crazy thing: many of my patients don't know that they have heart failure or that heart failure was the hospital's diagnosis of what happened to them and why they were being treated.

If your loved one was not on Lasix or water pills before, and they are on them now, then they very likely have a new diagnosis of heart failure. If they were given Lasix through an IV in the hospital or were told to increase the strength of their daily Lasix medication, then they were likely having a problem with heart failure when they were in the hospital.

The hospital chart has to designate the reasons that a person was admitted to the hospital and what they were treated for when they were there. There might be information on the discharge paperwork about their admitting or treating diagnoses, or there may be information sheets in the discharge paperwork about heart failure.

If you are unsure what the hospital wrote about why your loved one was there and what all was done while they were there, you can ask for a copy of your chart by calling the hospital's records department and requesting to have a copy printed. There is typically a small processing fee for this, but you need to know this information and have it for their records.

Your loved one's doctor can also request a copy of the paperwork from the hospital and can further explain to you what it says and what it means. If your loved one is in rehab, a nursing facility, outpatient therapy, or having home health care, their chart should also include referral information from the hospital, and you can ask them to look it over and help explain what it says.

Having heart failure does not mean that your loved one's heart has stopped working or that they are in immediate danger of dying. It does mean that their heart is not able to keep up with the demand being placed on it and that things can get very serious quickly if the doctor's instructions aren't followed.

Modern medicine has provided many supports to help manage this condition, but keeping heart failure under control requires a lot of commitment and understanding on the part of the patient and/or caregivers, and following the doctor's orders every single day.

Lasix (also known as "water pills" or "fluid pills"):

If the patient has been prescribed Lasix (water pills/fluid pills), they HAVE to take them as ordered. I hate that it makes them need to pee all the time, and I can fully appreciate how annoying and inconvenient that is, but if they don't release that extra fluid, their body will hold onto it, and this can lead to major problems.

Your heart is only designed to keep up with a certain amount of fluid circulating in your body. When your body starts holding onto fluid and swelling, it puts strain on your heart. If you have a diagnosis of heart failure already, your heart is not able to manage a normal amount of fluid on its own, much less more than a normal amount.

DO NOT let your loved one wait to take their fluid pill because they have things to do out of the house that day. Needing to run errands, having a doctor's appointment, and traveling are all NOT good excuses to skip or delay taking their pill.

Yes, it's really inconvenient to have to stop and go to the bathroom multiple times. Ending up in the hospital and paying all of those extra medical bills to go along with it is much more inconvenient. I promise!

If your loved one is on fluid pills and worried about leaks or accidents, they might need liners for their underwear or adult briefs. They do make adult briefs that are a lot more discreet these days. It might be necessary to pack a change of pants just in case.

At home, it might help to get a bedside commode for patients who are weak or easily worn out and are not complying with taking their Lasix because it's so difficult to get up and go to the bathroom so many times a day. For male patients, a hand urinal can also really up the convenience factor and help with compliance.

If the patient is on Lasix and also unable to walk at all or very much during the day, I would highly encourage you to put a barrier cream on their bottom to protect them from the moisture of urinating so frequently. The same way that you regularly put diaper cream on a baby because of constant exposure to urine, an adult who has leaks or uses adult briefs also likely needs something to protect their bottom.

If they do not have skin breakdown, and this is preventative, zinc oxide is a great option and can be found at any pharmacy. If you have been using a cream and they are still having a lot of redness or any amount of skin breakdown, their doctor needs to know about this right away and may need to prescribe something stronger to help prevent it from getting worse.

Weighing Daily:

If your loved one has heart failure, they need to weigh themselves every single day. This is extremely important for managing this condition because an unusual and sudden increase in weight is typically the first red flag that something is going wrong.

If the sudden weight gain is reported to the doctor immediately, this can almost always be treated at home or with a trip to the doctor's office. If the weight gain is unknown because the person is not weighing themselves daily, they can retain so much fluid that it becomes an emergency that requires hospitalization to fix.

If the person has a diagnosis of heart failure, they should have a cardiologist who is managing this condition. If they do not, get a referral from their primary doctor immediately. This is something that should be managed by a cardiologist.

Have a conversation with their cardiologist about tracking their weight and when to call the doctor's office. The standard practice is that a weight gain of two or more pounds overnight should be called in to the cardiologist's office.

Your loved one's doctor may have a different preference, and this could be for several reasons, including your loved one's medical history or other personal factors. You may be instructed to only call if the weight gain is 3+ pounds or maybe even four.

You may be instructed that if they gain a certain amount of weight, they need to go ahead and take a certain extra amount of their Lasix first, and then call in only if that doesn't bring them back to their normal weight by the end of the business day. You won't know until you ask the doctor, so it is very important to ask these questions.

The reason that checking weight daily helps with this is that it is not possible for the human body to gain 3 pounds of fat overnight. Eating a big meal the day before is not going to cause that change. But, your body can absolutely retain that much fluid overnight, and this is an early warning that the person's heart is having a much harder time than usual keeping up with their fluid levels. If this isn't addressed quickly, things can begin to tailspin.

If the person is only checking their weight once a week, let's say, they will not know if this weight gain happened slowly over a seven-day period or suddenly since the day before. Medically, there's a big difference between these two things, so weighing every single day is something that should not be skipped.

For the most consistency, weigh first thing in the morning, after using the bathroom, before eating, in the same type of clothes. Don't weigh in a light gown one morning, and fully dressed and wearing shoes the next.

What else do you need to know about this condition?

- Keeping the legs elevated as much as possible is very helpful for managing swelling. As a physical therapist, I want to clarify that the person needs to get up and walk throughout the day to maintain their strength and move their muscles, but if they are sitting, put those feet up!

- Compression stockings can be helpful for managing swelling too, but in this case, I would make sure to ask the doctor first if there is any reason that your loved one should not wear these. Sometimes there can be medical reasons that the doctor may not want them to wear compression stockings, so ask first.

- Most patients with heart failure are encouraged to follow a low sodium diet. If your loved one has not had a conversation with their doctor about their diet, please have this conversation. Low sodium does not simply mean to quit using the salt shaker. Sodium is used heavily in most preserved foods, like frozen and canned foods. Check the labels!

Nutrition Facts	
Valeur nutritive	
Per 1 cup (250 mL) / par 1 tasse (250 mL)	
Amount Teneur	% Daily Value % valeur quotidienne
Calories / Calories 80	
Fat / Lipides 0 g	0 %
Saturated / saturés 0 g + Trans / trans 0 g	0 %
Cholesterol / Cholestérol 0 mg	
Sodium / Sodium 115 mg	5 %
Carbohydrate / Glucides 12 g	4 %
Fibre / Fibres 0 g	0 %
Sugars / Sucres 11 g	
Protein / Protéines 9 g	
Vitamin A / Vitamine A	15 %
Vitamin C / Vitamine C	0 %
Calcium / Calcium	30 %
Iron / Fer	0 %
Vitamin D / Vitamine D	45 %

Amount of salt →

- In order to lower the amount of sodium in your loved one's diet, if they are limited in their food choices and do rely heavily on canned food, buy the cans that are labeled low sodium. Strain and rinse the food that comes in a can to remove most of the added salt.

- Many electrolyte drinks and supplements are high in salt too. Check the labels before assuming that these are a good option for your loved one.

- If your loved one is on a fluid restriction, keep in mind that all fluids count. This includes coffee, tea, Popsicles, soup broth, ice cream, etc.

- Make sure and have a conversation with the cardiologist about whether or not the patient needs to be on a fluid restriction, and how much of a restriction. The standard amount is 2000 mL of fluid per day. Patients with more advanced heart failure may be reduced to a 1500 mL per day restriction.

- If you find that managing daily weight is very difficult or fluctuates a lot, go back and look at sodium levels, and how much fluid the person is taking in each day. Have a conversation with the cardiologist about your concerns.

Heart Attack

Heart attack - If your loved one had a heart attack that caused them to be admitted to the hospital, chances are very high that their blood pressure medication was changed while they were there. Here is a chart to help you understand high and low blood pressures:

Blood Pressure Category	Top Number (Systolic)	Bottom Number (Diastolic)	What to do? (Always check that blood pressure meds have been taken.)
Dangerously High	180+	110+	Call 911 or report to emergency room immediately.
Too High	160-179	100-109	Call PCP or Cardiologist for instructions. If no answer or call back, call 911.
High	140-159	85-99	Call PCP or cardiologist for instructions. Set up an appointment to come in. Watch stress and diet.
Normal	90-139	60-84	Good job!
Too Low	80-89	50-59	Call PCP or cardiologist for instructions. Set up an appointment to come in. Watch for signs of dehydration.
Dangerously Low	Less than 80	Less than 50	Call 911 or report to emergency room immediately.

I cannot stress enough how important it is to:

- Monitor the patient's blood pressure and symptoms after they get home.

- Complete the medication section of this book so that you are crystal clear on which medications your loved one should be taking.

- Follow up with their primary doctor and specialists about any medication changes that were made in the hospital.

- Pay attention to, and report, any unusual symptoms including exhaustion, lightheadedness, dizziness, feeling faint, etc. along with reporting blood pressure readings that are too high or too low.

Make sure you take your loved one's blood pressure every day, and keep track of these readings. If you would like a great resource to track and organize vital signs, I made a logbook just for you, "Track Your Loved One's Vital Signs." You can get a copy at www.helpthecaregiver.com/store. This logbook also has more information about taking and interpreting blood pressure, so it's a great resource.

In home health, I have seen many instances of patients who were sent home with too many blood pressure medications after having a heart attack. They get home and feel weak, tired, and like they might pass out. When I take their blood pressure, I get a very low reading.

If your loved one is complaining of dizziness or lightheadedness, please read the chapter on dizziness. The second half of that chapter is focused on blood pressure.

If the patient has low blood pressure, the doctor needs to be called right away. They will need to know what blood pressure medication the patient is taking, how strong the dose is for each medication, and any symptoms the patient is having related to lightheadedness, dizziness, nausea, feeling faint, headache, etc.

Please do not stop taking a blood pressure medication without calling the doctor first. Some medications are going to lower blood pressure, but they might also be addressing other heart-related issues that the person is having, such as afib or to control their heart rate.

It's not safe to suddenly stop taking any medication, so call the doctor's office and leave a message for the nurse. They should get back to you very quickly.

It's important to track and report unusual symptoms. Only some heart attacks come with the stereotypical chest pain and/or radiating pain down your arm. And this is even less likely to be the case for women. Sometimes a heart attack can show itself as extreme nausea, throwing up for several days, unrelenting headache, unusual fatigue, etc.

Also, please be aware that the same person can have very different symptoms with each different heart attack. The symptoms they had with the first one might not be the same symptoms they have with others.

If your loved one has a personal history or a family history of heart issues (their sibling, parents, or grandparents had a lot of problems with their heart or a history of heart attacks), then you need to pay attention and take action if the person has concerning symptoms. The faster a heart attack can be helped by a medical team, the less damage that will usually be done.

If you think that your loved one is potentially having an issue with their heart, please report to the ER. Call an ambulance if you need to. If they are not having chest pain, but you still think it might be a heart problem, you need to tell any medical person who will listen that you are worried that it's their heart.

If there is any concern at all that your loved one might be having a heart attack, they will do an EKG on them. They'll even check this in the waiting room of the emergency room if they have to, but they are going to check that before they do anything else. It's that time-sensitive and that important!

However, if your loved one insists that they are probably fine, it's probably nothing, it's just nausea, etc., it could take a very long time before anyone checks their heart, and by that point, a lot of damage can be done.

COPD

COPD - Chronic Obstructive Pulmonary Disease (pulmonary = lung) is a very stressful problem to have. Whether this was the reason your loved one was in the hospital in the first place, or if it is a disease that they are also managing, this section will have valuable information.

COPD is exhausting and can be overwhelming. It's scary to not be able to breathe or catch your breath! It's also hard to have any energy left when you're spending so much of the energy you do have managing your breathing.

Many patients with COPD are also smokers. I am not going to tell a patient to stop smoking. They know the risks, they've been told a million times, and me telling them to stop is not going to make a difference.

What I WILL encourage my patients to do is to try to cut back on how much they are smoking each day. Every puff on a cigarette causes damage. Any reduction in the amount of smoking is a win. Going from a full pack a day to a half a pack a day is still a win.

I had a friend once who weaned herself off of cigarettes by smoking only a half of a cigarette every time she went to smoke. The frequency and habit of smoking at certain time points during the day was a very hard habit to break, but she found that she was able to stop smoking the cigarette at the halfway point and then finish it the next time she went for a break.

I have had many patients who have used this method to successfully pull back on the amount of cigarettes they smoke, and I celebrate the heck out of that accomplishment.

A person is not going to be able to stop smoking until they are ready, and some people are just not interested in changing that habit. We can get frustrated about it, or we can make peace with it, but they are the only ones who can decide that for themselves and hold to their decision.

I have seen some family members who are caring for very sick loved ones who continuously end up in the hospital due to breathing problems eventually get to the point where they refuse to buy cigarettes for their loved one. They are done enabling a bad habit, and if the patient is not physically able to get to the store to buy the cigarettes for themselves, the caregiver is actually more in control of that habit than the patient. I won't tell you to do that, but I have seen many caregivers get to that point.

Here are the biggest things to keep in mind with this condition:

- If your loved one has been prescribed an inhaler, it is very important for them to have a healthcare professional, either a doctor, a nurse, a therapist, etc., watch them demonstrate using this inhaler. I cannot tell you the staggering number of patients I have seen who either didn't use an inhaler because they didn't know how, or were convinced that they did know how to use one, but they were actually using it wrong.

- I know it is so frustrating for the patient, but they have to respect the limits that they have with their breathing. They cannot power through an inability to breathe. When the breathing is getting too heavy, the person absolutely must sit down and take a break until their breathing has slowed back down. Slow and steady wins here.

- Physical and occupational therapy can be an amazing combination for someone with COPD. Physical therapy typically focuses on building strength and endurance in order to allow someone to be able to do more than they could do before through normal ways, like cooking while standing up.

- Occupational therapy can help problem-solve a lot of creative ways that a person can do a task differently than usual, in a way that is not nearly as tiring for them, such as cooking while sitting down or planning to take sitting breaks during meal prep. This is generally referred to as energy conservation training, and I highly recommend it for my patients with COPD.

- COPD is a condition where the lungs are essentially overinflated all of the time, which means that it is very difficult to breathe all of the air that is in your lungs out. Breathing in through the nose and out through pursed lips (the way you would blow out a candle) can be very helpful for managing breathing because it gives more time to ease the trapped air out.

Gently remind your loved one to breathe in through their nose and out through their mouth when they seem out of breath.

- Talking uses a lot of oxygen. If your loved one is a talker, and you are noticing that they are breathing very fast and having a hard time catching their breath, gently encourage them to take a minute to focus on their breathing before finishing what they are trying to say.

- Air quality in the home can make a huge difference in someone's ability to breathe easily when they have COPD. One thing I see in home health a lot is tons of pet hair. If there is visible pet hair on the floor, furniture, or bedding of a person's home with COPD, that has to be cleaned up and kept away! It IS making it harder for them to breathe.

- The same with thick layers of dust; this has to be cleaned up and maintained. It is extremely difficult for a person to manage their breathing otherwise. Investing in an air purifier or automatic vacuum can be a great option and is significantly cheaper than another trip to the hospital.

- Secondhand smoke from other people in the home who use cigarettes or vape pens can have a negative effect on someone's ability to breathe when they have COPD. If anyone in the home is smoking indoors, the rules need to change to insist that all smoking will be done outside to protect the air quality in the home.

If the person is on oxygen:

- If your loved one is on oxygen, they should NOT take their oxygen off when they get up to move around. It takes MORE oxygen to keep up with your body's needs when you are moving. If they need the oxygen while resting, they need it even more when they are up!

- If they're taking the oxygen line off because it won't reach the bathroom or wherever they are trying to go, get an extension for the oxygen line (either by calling the company who provided the oxygen machine and asking for an extension line or by purchasing one online). Some patients leave the extension on all the time. Others prefer to add the extension when they need to get up and take it back off once they are settled back in their chair. Either way is fine.

- Another option is to move the oxygen machine to a more central location between the rooms so that it will reach both areas.

- Oxygen lines pose a tripping hazard! Please encourage your loved one to move more carefully than usual and to keep their eye on the oxygen line and where their feet are to lower their chances of tripping and falling.

- Oxygen also poses an explosion hazard. Be mindful to keep all gas and sparks away from the oxygen tank and the part of the oxygen line that goes into the person's nose. No hairspray, cigarettes, vapes, matches, gas for the stove, propane tanks, open flames, or fires.

- Have a gas stove? Keep the oxygen and the person wearing it out of the kitchen while the stove is on.

- Does someone in the home smoke? Not around the oxygen tanks or lines. If the person must smoke, the safest place to do that is outside. If the patient is the one who smokes, they need to go outside away from the oxygen. Taking the oxygen line off will make it harder to breathe, but it is significantly better than risking an explosion on the person's face.

- If the person was sent home on oxygen for the first time, it's possible that their need for it is only temporary. Just because they were sent home on oxygen does not mean that the doctor had the intention of them using it forever, but they demonstrated a need to have it at that time.

- You may have seen a lot of commercials on tv about portable oxygen that can be carried with a shoulder strap when leaving the house. It is important to know that there are strict guidelines that must be met for patients to qualify for insurance to cover one of these. The patient must have been on oxygen for several months in a row (typically 3) and go through several tanks of oxygen each month (I've seen quotes of 8 tanks per month) and need the oxygen around the clock. Some people will pay out of pocket for these if insurance will not cover the cost, but they are several thousand dollars and only some companies provide the ability to purchase one without insurance.

- As a physical therapist, I have helped many patients to wean off of oxygen when it was appropriate and in a way that was safe. Trying to wean off of oxygen yourself without any instructions or guidance from a professional can be very dangerous. If this is one of your loved one's goals, have a conversation with their doctor about this desire, and get a referral to therapy or pulmonary rehab if appropriate.

Pneumonia

Pneumonia - I absolutely hate to see my patients suffering from hospitalization due to pneumonia. It's so miserable and so exhausting, and very scary because it often makes it so hard to breathe.

One of the biggest keys to getting rid of pneumonia and keeping it from coming back is the way the person is breathing. Let's talk about some key information that I give to my patients every single time I admit one to home health for pneumonia.

When you breathe in air, the oxygen comes into your lungs and passes through your lungs into your bloodstream. This is how you get lots of fresh oxygen to the body. If your lungs are sick from a pneumonia infection, that infection is making it harder for the lungs to work like they should because the infection is blocking the passage of oxygen through the lungs.

If you are only taking tiny, quick breaths, you are barely taking in enough oxygen to keep the body going, and your body will stay tired and sick. It can make it feel like you are constantly gasping for air and can't get in a full breath.

This is the analogy I use for breathing: let's say you have a thick, dry sponge, and a bucket of water. If you lightly tap that sponge on the surface of the water and quickly pull it back, there will be a little bit of water on the sponge, but the sponge will definitely not be full of water.

However, if you leave the sponge on the water and give it more time, it will absorb more and more of the water and eventually become soaking wet. This is how sick lungs work with breathing in air.

Breathing tiny little breaths is like tapping that sponge on the top of the water and then being surprised that it's not soaking wet. If you can take a slow, deep breath, that will help to get more and more of the oxygen into your body, the way that letting the sponge sit in the water will cause it to become soaked. Focus on slower, deeper breathing to really catch your breath.

Pneumonia is an infection that is in your lungs and has created a thick coating of mucus that is blocking your lungs from working normally. In order to get rid of the infection completely, you have to break up that infection and mucus and get it out of your lungs; otherwise, it will just stay there and make you sicker.

Here's the other analogy I use: let's say you have a little fishbowl full of ocean water with sand at the bottom. If you only splash at the top of the water, you might get a little bit of movement from some of the sand, but mostly the sand will stay settled at the bottom of the bowl. If you want to kick up that sand, you have to reach all the way down into the bottom of the bowl.

One of the very best ways to break up and get rid of a pneumonia infection is with deep breathing. Usually, the infection settles at the bottom of your lungs, the way sand does in a fishbowl. Taking tiny shallow breaths is the same thing as splashing at the top of the fishbowl. You will never reach what's at the bottom of the bowl that way.

Taking strong, deep breaths has the same effect as reaching down to the bottom of the fishbowl to break up the sand at the bottom. That's why so many of the exercises patients are given when they have pneumonia are related to breathing as deeply as possible and increasing how much they can breathe.

With all of that in mind, here are the top things to pay attention to when recovering from pneumonia:

- Have your loved one use the breathing device that they were given at the hospital as much as they possibly can during the day. This will help make their breathing stronger. If for some reason they were not given one of these devices, I strongly recommend that you get one. You can find my recommendation on my website helpthecaregiver.com/store or search on Amazon for "incentive spirometer."

- Have them focus on taking deep breaths as much as possible through-out the day. This will help their lungs get stronger, but it will also help them feel like they are able to catch their breath.

- Cough big and loud! Do not hold back on coughing. Coughing is the body's natural way to help force all of that junk from the pneumonia out of their lungs, but only if it is a big strong cough. If my patients ever apologize for coughing, I tell them I want them to cough even bigger and louder. Take a deep breath in (remember the sand??) and a big strong cough out.

- Do NOT give them cough suppressants. Don't give medication of any kind to stop them from coughing. I know that the coughing is aggravating and can create a lot of discomfort in their chest, but this is the body's natural way of getting rid of this infection, and we need to encourage it as much as possible.

- Finish the antibiotic. Even if the person feels completely better, take every last pill! Just because they feel better does not mean that the infection has completely cleared up. It might only mean that the infection has cleared up to the point that it is not bothering them anymore, but it is still there. If the antibiotic clears up some, but not all, of the infection, the infection can come back stronger the next time, and it might be resistant to that antibiotic now.

- If the patient feels like they are starting to get worse again, do not wait. Go to urgent care (not the hospital) to request a chest x-ray to see if the infection is still there or getting worse. Urgent care can take care of this quickly and easily if it is addressed in the early stages. If you wait until it is an emergency, you're very likely looking at another hospitalization.

- You can also call the patient's doctor to let them know what is going on and the concern that the pneumonia is coming back, but most doctors' offices are not going to be able to do a same-day x-ray. They are likely going to tell you to report to urgent care and have the results of the x-ray sent to them.

- It's also a great idea to both go to urgent care and call the patient's doctor to let them know what is going on. If the x-ray does not show infection, the doctor may still want them to come in for a check-up. If that is the case, make it a top priority to get in as soon as possible to find out why the patient is feeling so bad.

Orthopedic Surgeries

I have many patients in home health who are fresh out of these surgeries, and I want to address some key points related to them.

A few reminders first:

If your loved one **had to have this surgery because of an injury from a fall, please make sure to read the sections on home safety, medications, dizziness, and falls** to prevent another fall that could cause them to end up back in the hospital.

Anytime there is a **surgical wound, there is potential for infection.** Please refer to the **section in this chapter about preventing surgical infections** for more information.

Anyone who has had **surgery is at an increased risk for a blood clot.** Please refer to the **section about blood clots** for more information.

After surgery, it is common for someone to be **prescribed medication for pain.** Please see the **section about pain medication** for further information.

Total Hip Replacement

- The patient will be on hip precautions after the surgery. Which hip precautions they are on will depend on whether the incision site is on the front of the hip or the back. Make sure you are clear about which precautions the surgeon wants the patient to follow.

- It is standard for these hip precautions to be in place until the patient is 12 weeks out from surgery. Yes, that is three months! If you need clarification, ask the surgeon. If the surgeon has not designated a different time frame, then assume that the patient is under these restrictions for 12 weeks from the date of the surgery.

- The reason for these precautions has to do with the way the hip works and is shaped. Directly after this surgery, the hip is at a higher risk of dislocating. It's very important to not put the hip at extreme angles that could cause this dislocation to happen.

- However, I really want to emphasize that as long as the precautions are followed, the chances of that complication happening are extremely small. I have had several patients who have been scared to the point that they refused to move out of fear of dislocating their hip after the surgery. Please don't feel that this is a likely outcome unless your loved one has a personal history that puts them at a much higher risk than the normal population for this complication.

- A freshly replaced hip will tell you in real-time (meaning, it will hurt right away) when you have hit a limit and need to take a break. As long as your loved one listens to their body and takes a break when the hip starts hurting, they will have very well-managed pain and should have a smooth and easy recovery.

- Attempting to push through pain on a freshly replaced hip is a very bad idea and will cause a lot of unnecessary discomfort. They can move around until the hip tells them to stop. Have them take a break until they are well-rested. Repeat. It really is that straightforward with a hip replacement!

- If the person is doing a great job of listening to their body and taking breaks, they may have little to no pain at all. I love it when that happens! If that is the case, no one needs to push them to take their pain pills. Honestly, if they say they don't need a pain pill, they don't.

- Ice is great to manage swelling. NO heat to the area until 6-8 weeks out from the surgery, because heat can increase swelling in a new surgical area, and that can actually cause more discomfort.

Total Knee Replacement

All about pain after this surgery:

- Pain management is the biggest thing on everyone's mind after a total knee replacement. Once a freshly replaced knee moves into high levels of pain, it can be extremely difficult to get the pain under control.

- For specific instructions and precautions about pain pills in general, please refer to that section below.

- Stay in front of the pain. Try not to let the pain get above a 7 on a 0 to 10 scale. If the pain is climbing and gets to a seven, do something about it. Taking a pain pill or applying ice will still take a little while to kick in. If you delay taking action, the pain will be so high by the time action is taken that it won't help very much.

- Day 3 after surgery is typically when the pain is the highest. Things should start to get a little more manageable after that, and if they don't, contact the surgeon.

- Pain after a total knee replacement has a big delay. As opposed to a freshly replaced hip, which will tell the person right away if they are doing too much, a knee will lie to you. A person can be walking around the house and thinking that they are feeling great and doing well, and then, four hours later, the pain hits like a truck, and now the person realizes they overdid it, but it's too late to do anything about it.

- When it comes to activity after a knee replacement, the person should go slow and take it easy. Do a little bit one day. If they wake up the next day and did not have any major increase in their pain, add 10% more activity over the course of the whole next day. Repeat. This is how to build up activity without triggering major pain cycles. Slow and steady wins the race on this one!

- Because pain after this surgery can be tricky, please do not let your loved one be in a hurry to get off the pain pills! They can be a hero about something else. This isn't the time. If they are genuinely not hurting, then delay taking a pain pill until the pain reaches that seven out of 10 that we talked about. Otherwise, have them take a pain pill before going to bed and before doing physical therapy as a bare minimum for the first 2-3 weeks.

- Last word about pain here: I have so many patients that tell me they are going to push through the pain after this surgery. Sometimes you just have to let a person get miserable before they will listen, but here is what I will tell my extra stubborn patients when I can see that this is going to be a problem: "you literally just had a surgical bandsaw cut off the end of your thigh bone and your shin bone. The surgeon then took a very fancy mallet and press-fitted your new knee into those same bones by banging on that component like a construction worker hammering nails through a 2 x 4. You can't push through that. There is no amount of stubbornness that is going to allow your body to heal faster than it can from that kind of trauma. Just take the pain pills and rest when you need to!"

Everything else to know about recovering from a total knee replacement:

- It's very common for there to be a huge delay in bruising after this surgery. If the person wakes up on day five and finds that their leg is suddenly bruised from hip to toe, it's not actually going to surprise the surgeon. If there isn't any increase in pain to go with it, it's nothing to worry about.

- Absolutely no lotion, vitamin E oil, etc., on or immediately around the incision site. We want a strong, tight recovery of the skin. Skin is like paper; it's already not the toughest thing in the world, and if it gets wet, it's even more likely to tear. The surgical site needs to get dry and crusty to protect itself. Don't pick the scab.

- If the patient has been sent home with a surgical bandage, and that bandage has become dark with blood, the surgeon needs to be contacted. You absolutely cannot let a bandage that is saturated with blood sit on a fresh surgical wound. That is a recipe for infection!

- I don't mean little spots of blood, but if more than 30% of the bandage is dark, go ahead and call the nurse's line and ask for instructions. Take a picture if you need to be able to send it to the surgeon or nurse. Do not wait. If it's the weekend, call the on-call line!

- There is a ton of swelling in the knee and after a knee replacement, and the swelling is one of the top reasons for the amount of pain after this surgery. Keep ice on your knee and leg around the clock to manage swelling and pain. You cannot use too much ice, and it's fine to sleep with ice on the area. For extra relief, put ice underneath the knee too.

- It's normal for there to be swelling in the calf and foot after this surgery. Any increase in calf tenderness or overall swelling in the leg should be reported to the surgeon. Otherwise, it should not be anything to worry about. If the surgeon has prescribed compression stockings, this can help manage the swelling. Keeping the foot up when resting will also help. For more guidance, see the section coming up on blood clots.

- If they sent you home with one of those ice machines, thank your lucky stars. You can freeze plastic water bottles to put in the cooling compartment instead of using ice to save the money and hassle of using so much ice so quickly. Fill it up right before you go to sleep and sleep with it running.

- I know that moving the knee is extremely uncomfortable, especially in the first few days. However, a knee that isn't moving will stiffen up very quickly which can lead to bad outcomes. It is incredibly important to move the knee frequently after surgery. Have the person ease into it, take their time, and take breaks when they need to; just keep that knee moving.

- When they tell you not to put a pillow under the knee after surgery, they mean not to put it in such a way that encourages the need to bend. If you need to put a pillow under the entire leg so that it is under the calf and thigh as well, this is perfectly fine to do if it helps with comfort or elevating the foot to help with swelling.

- No one should be in a hurry to walk with a cane after a knee replacement. The person is ready to walk with a cane when they can do so without a limp. If they use the cane before they are ready, they will be practicing walking around with a limp, and that will become their new normal walking pattern. They didn't go through all of this to come out on the other side with a limp! Encourage them to take their time getting off of the walker. Better a few extra weeks with a walker than a lifetime of limping that will eventually lead to hip and/or back pain.

Back Surgery

There can be a lot of questions and worries after a person has had back surgery. I want to go over a few things that I find myself repeating to a lot of patients after they've come home from back surgery, regardless of what type of back surgery they have had.

Pain with this surgery:

It can be very normal for the person to be in as much or more pain for 6 to 8 weeks after the surgery as they were in before the surgery. This does not mean that the surgery didn't work.

If they had surgery because something in their back was pressing on something else, either a disk out of place, a narrowing of the spinal canal, swelling, a pinched nerve, etc., then the surgeon corrected this, but the body's natural swelling response to having surgery basically replaces the pressure that was there in the first place.

Once the natural swelling in the body goes away, then the person will be able to know what the surgery was truly able to fix. Please try not to stress or worry about the surgery being a failure. The person won't know the full effect that the surgery had until they are out of this initial healing phase.

It is also very normal for a patient to have a confusing amount of pain in their hip or thigh after back surgery. This can be due to the way the patient had to be placed and secured onto the surgical table in order to allow the surgeon to do the surgery.

It's one of those little things that many surgeons don't think to warn you about, but often a little bit of massage and a heating pad can go a long way towards managing this discomfort.

The same way that a newly replaced hip will tell the person right away when they are doing too much, the back will be the same. As long as the person stops and takes a break when they start feeling an increase in back pain, their pain should be very well managed. Trying to push and push and push once the hurting starts is what will get a person into trouble.

If the person is not hurting and doesn't want to take their pain pills, that's fine. Their body will tell them immediately when to stop doing something, and as long as they listen to that, they really should not be getting into high levels of pain that cannot be controlled.

Other things to keep in mind with back surgery:

- If the person has numbness in their legs or feet, they are at very high risk for falls and need to take extra caution when getting up or walking.

- If the person has been put on spinal precautions, think of a BLT sandwich. No Bending, Lifting, or Twisting. Spinal precautions should be followed for 12 weeks following the date of the surgery, unless stated otherwise by the surgeon. If you aren't sure if your loved one is supposed to be on spinal precautions, call the surgeon's office and ask.

- If the person was given a surgical back brace to wear, it is expected that this brace also needs to be worn for 12 weeks after the date of the surgery, unless stated otherwise by the surgeon.

- I know that back braces can be extremely uncomfortable and difficult to take on and off multiple times throughout the day. It only has to be snugly fit when the person is standing or moving around. I have convinced many patients to wear their brace by showing them to loosen the side straps while they are sitting and then tighten them when they go to stand. This keeps them compliant with the brace and makes it much more comfortable to wear when sitting, without the hassle of taking it on and off so many times.

- The brace does not need to be worn when the person is sleeping at night. It is meant to protect them when they are moving from doing things that can aggravate the spine or surgery site.

- If a person is having a hard time complying with their post-surgical instructions, I will explain to them that the problem with not minding their precautions or not wearing their brace is that every time they move in the wrong way, they are aggravating the part of their spine that is trying to heal. It's like picking a scab over and over. The healing gets to a certain point, and then you pick at it until it bleeds, and now your body has gone two steps back and has to start again with the healing process. Healing your spine can be the same way. The body can heal the area to a point, but if you are constantly doing things that aggravate the healing process, it causes your body to go two steps back and take that much longer to heal.

Preventing Infection After Surgery

The big fear on everyone's mind after surgery is the potential for infection. Anytime there is surgery, a wound, or other opening on the body that is new, there is a potential for bacteria to get in and cause an infection. Let's talk about how to prevent it and what to look for.

Sometimes the surgeon will have the patient take antibiotics as a preventative measure. If antibiotics have been prescribed, make sure they are taken as directed until the last one is gone! Do not stop them early.

The patient needs a clean environment to minimize their chance for infection. The sheets on their bed need to be clean. If they get dirty from a bowl or bladder accident, blood, food being spilled, or pet dander, the sheets need to be changed.

If their favorite chair is old, dirty, or covered in food or pet hair, place a clean towel, sheet, or other barrier between the part of their body that had the surgery and the chair.

If the wound is on their foot, they do not need to walk around the house barefoot. Even if the floors have been mopped and the carpet has been vacuumed, there could be something at any point that could transfer from the floor to the wound on their foot and cause a problem.

A light protective shoe, a post-surgical walking boot, or a wrap, bandage, or sock needs to be worn. If what they are wearing is cloth, it needs to be changed and cleaned frequently to avoid absorbing dirt or fluid and holding it against the wound.

If the covering gets wet, either from stepping in something or because the wound has leaked or bled, the covering must be changed immediately. Under no circumstances should a wet or soiled covering be allowed to be held against a wound.

Caring for the wound itself:

- Moisture held against the body is a breeding ground for skin breakdown and infection. If the person has a post-surgical bandage or wound dressing, and you notice that it seems very moist from any bodily fluid, including sweat, urine, or blood, the surgeon needs to be contacted right away about what needs to be done to change that dressing or bandage.

- I don't care if the instructions say to leave everything in place for seven days and then remove whatever dressing is there. Those instructions assume that the wound is not saturated or dirty. Do not remove anything without instructions from the surgeon, but also do not let this go unreported. Take pictures, insist on coming into the doctor's office if you need to, but do not let a dirty or saturated bandage sit on a person's skin for several days.

- If the person has incontinence of the bowel or bladder, meaning that they are not able to make it to the bathroom in time when they need to pee or poop, and they use the bathroom in such a way that some of that pee or poop gets on a surgical wound or dressing, the doctor needs to be alerted to this as soon as it happens or as soon as you are aware of it.

- If your loved one was sent home with a surgical dressing or bandage, and you are unclear about when that dressing is supposed to be removed, let's get clear about it. Look at the discharge paperwork first. Most of the time, there will be instructions somewhere in that information packet that will say when the dressing is supposed to be removed. It might be something you are expected to do at home, or it could be something that the surgeon is planning to do when the patient comes in for a follow-up visit.

- If you don't see an answer on the discharge papers, please call the surgeon's office and ask what you are supposed to do about the bandage. Do you leave it on until the patient comes in for the post-op visit? Is it supposed to be taken off after a certain number of days? Again, leaving this on too long can cause problems, so don't just assume the surgeon's intentions.

Animals and the risk for infection or complications:

- Do not let animals near a fresh incision site. I can fully appreciate a loving relationship with a cat or dog, and I absolutely understand that they probably missed the patient while they were gone to have the surgery, but they can unintentionally cause infection by scratching at the person near the surgery site and making just enough of a puncture in the skin to let infection in.

- Their pet hair, even if they have recently been bathed, can pose an increased risk for infection if it gets on or in the surgery site. Cats and dogs do not need to lay on a surgery site or post-surgical bandages or dressings.

- Cats or dogs that are insistent about jumping onto the patient while they are sitting in a recliner or on their bed must be controlled in such a way to keep them from doing this. They might have to be gated up in another room for a few days. They might need to be physically blocked from the patient's chair for a few days. They might need to be on a leash inside that is being held by another family member. I know that can feel stressful for the patient and the animal, but having the person end up back in the hospital because of an infection will be more traumatic for both of them.

- Do not let an animal lick a wound. I have seen several patients who allow this to happen for one reason or another. It should never happen under any circumstances. I don't care if the person feels that the animal is trying to help. I don't care if they have heard an old wives' tale that there's something beneficial in the animal's mouth that will help (there isn't). It is 100% a huge risk for infection and should absolutely not be allowed.

- If an animal is one that likes to jump on the patient or scratch at them for attention, these behaviors need to be limited after the person has just had surgery. They are less steady on their feet, and less able to react to being jumped on, which puts them at a higher risk for falls. Also, the scratching or just the sharpness of the animal's nails when jumping up on a person can create small scratches on the skin that can become an entrance point for bacteria and infection.

Red flags for infection:

It can be difficult to know if what you're looking at is normal after surgery or if it is an indication that an infection is starting. Here are some general guidelines for assessing a wound for infection and when to report certain symptoms.

As always, please have a conversation with the surgeon about anything in particular that they want you to look for and report as a potential complication after the surgery.

- **Color:** Surgery will create discoloration. It's normal for an incision site to have changes in color after the surgery. It can be a good idea to take pictures of the surgical site early on for comparison. If the redness or discoloration increases significantly, especially if the discoloration looks like a streaking pattern away from the surgical site, this can be a red flag.

- **Heat:** It is also normal for a new surgical site to feel warm. However, there is a difference between the skin feeling warm and feeling like it's on fire. If the heat seems extreme or if there is a large increase in heat compared to normal, this can be a red flag. Some people's bodies run warmer than others, so check the opposite side of the body for comparison.

- **Pain:** The key here is a sudden increase in pain that was not there before. Surgeries are going to hurt, and different people have different pain tolerances. It's normal for a person to have a high level of pain in the first few days after the surgery. If the pain has not backed off at all by day four after the surgery, there could be many reasons for that, but the surgeon needs to be called. If the person is three weeks out from their surgery and their pain has been running at about 5 out of 10 on average, and they wake up one morning with their pain at an 8 or 9 out of 10, that is a big red flag and needs to be reported to the doctor immediately.

- **Swelling:** Some surgeries naturally cause more swelling than others. Swelling after a total knee replacement can go on for months, while there is usually little to no visible signs of swelling after a shoulder surgery. So again, we are comparing how the person is doing now to how they have been doing in the previous several days. If they have been having a medium amount of swelling up to this point, and they are suddenly having a very large amount of swelling, this can be a red flag.

With swelling and pain, pay attention to the person's activity levels. A lot of times, I will have a patient who is starting to feel better after their surgery, so they immediately go out and try to do all the things they haven't been able to do for months. They clean the whole house, walk around the entire block, and spend the day running errands. The next morning, they wake up swollen and in a ton of pain. If there seems to be an obvious answer for these changes that is directly related to overdoing it with activity, then it is not likely to be an infection.

However, a sudden increase in redness, especially accompanied by streaking discoloration in a starburst pattern or straight line pattern away from the incision, requires an immediate call to the doctor's office, no matter what other symptoms or what level of activity the person has experienced. (See picture below)

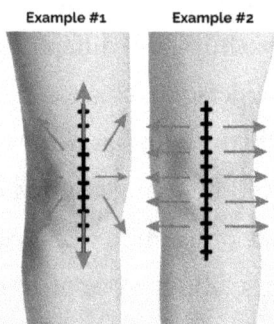

If there is an infection, it can typically be taken care of at home with the surgeon calling in antibiotics. It becomes an emergency when it is ignored. An infection that has been ignored will spread. When it spreads, it can become necessary to be hospitalized to get it under control. It's much better to speak up early on the off chance it turns out to be "nothing" than to wait until it is too late.

Blood Clots

A blood clot is a very serious and very dangerous potential complication after surgery. Many times, a patient will be given medication to prevent a blood clot if they have had surgery. The medication could be a baby aspirin, or it might be something stronger like Eliquis.

Make sure you are aware of the surgeon's instructions when it comes to taking this medication for blood clot prevention. I've seen too many instances where the patient was given instructions at the hospital but, after coming home, realized they were very unsure about when to stop taking the blood clot prevention medication or when to go back to their old medication routine.

If the patient was on a daily aspirin before the surgery, they may have been instructed to keep taking it by itself, to keep taking it and also take something else like Eliquis, or to stop taking the aspirin and replace it with Eliquis.

Which of these were the instructions for your loved one? If you are not sure, it probably says on the discharge paperwork that was sent home with them. If you cannot find it on the discharge paperwork, call the surgeon's office and ask.

If their blood clot medication routine was changed, how long are they supposed to go by this new change? Until their follow-up appointment with the surgeon? For 7, 14, or 30 days? Until the Eliquis runs out, and then do they go back to normal? If you are unsure, check the discharge instructions. If you cannot find specific instructions, call the surgeon's office and ask. It's very important that everyone is clear when it comes to blood clot prevention medication instructions.

The best thing a person can do to prevent a blood clot, along with following the medication instructions from the surgeon, is to move. Move the body part that had the surgery, get up and walk if possible. Have them do ankle pumps like they're obsessed with them. Keeping the blood circulating will significantly lower the chance of it clotting.

How often should a person do ankle pumps? As often as they can think about it. The more, the better. How often should a person get up to move? The ideal answer here is once an hour. The realistic answer is that multiple times a day should be enough.

What are the red flags of a potential blood clot? Blood clots usually happen in the calf, upper thigh/groin, or inner upper arm, with the calf being the most common. If your loved one feels a high level of unusual pain in one of these areas, especially if it is very tender to the touch or the person jumps with pain when someone applies light pressure to the area, they need to be checked for a blood clot. Call the surgeon (if they have just had a surgery), or their PCP or cardiologist to report the symptoms and tell them you are concerned about a possible blood clot.

The surgeon or other doctor may tell the person to come into their office, or have them go to a local urgent care office to have an ultrasound done of the area. An ultrasound is painless but the only way to verify whether or not a person has a blood clot.

If the person is having the tenderness and swelling in one of these areas and also starts having chest pain, trouble with breathing, or a headache that is unusual for them, that needs to be seen about right away. This could be an indication of a blood clot that has traveled and become an emergency, so call 911 or report to the emergency room.

Pain Medication

We've covered when to take the pain pills for knee, back, and hip surgeries in the related sections above. Here are a few more tips for taking pain pills and potential side effects from them.

- Keep in mind that besides a traditional pain pill after surgery, such as oxycodone, the patient may also be taking other medications, like aspirin for clot prevention, gabapentin for nerve pain, and anti-spasm medication. All of these will have a pain-relieving effect, so I always recommend to my patients to spread out when these are being taken. It's better to take a little bit of something every two or three hours for pain instead of taking a whole lot of pain medication at once and then having to wait 6 to 8 hours to take anything else.

- Many pain pills can make a person drowsy. Someone who is drowsy is at a higher risk of falling, so please be extra careful when changing positions and walking. If the drowsiness is frustrating to the person, try only taking half of a pill or spreading out when the different medications are being taken to make sure they're not getting too many pain relieving medications at the same time.

- Strong pain pills can cause constipation. Constipation can become a full-blown emergency if it goes on for too long. If it has been at least three days since the patient has had a full bowel movement, it's time to take something to help that process along. Start with something gentle like a stool softener, and work your way up from there.

- Keep in mind that stool softeners can have a 12 to 48-hour delay in their effect. Don't start taking a ton of things all at once. Take something and then give it at least 12 hours before considering taking something else. This is also why it's important to go ahead and take something if it's been three days, because even if you start taking something, it can be a while before that medication works.

- If the person is allergic to pain pills or unable to take them due to extreme nausea or constipation, have a conversation with the surgeon to see if he or she would be willing to prescribe an alternative to manage their pain instead. I have seen gabapentin and anti-spasm medication do wonders for pain management after orthopedic surgeries.

- Please note that it is against the law (in many, if not all states) to drive while on narcotic level pain pills. If a person were to get into an accident and there was suspicion that the person was "under the influence," and it was found that the person had these pills in their system, they could get a DUI. It has happened many times in the areas where I have worked, so please don't let your loved one take that risk.

- Don't only rely on pain pills for pain management. Controlling a person's swelling can do just as much for post-surgical pain as the pain pills do. Having a therapist or someone else do a little bit of massage on an extremely tight muscle can also do wonders. Ice and elevation! Making sure to keep a balance between getting up and moving and not overdoing it are key elements to pain management.

UTI – "Urinary Tract Infection"

Many of my older patients are hospitalized due to urinary tract infections. Hospitalization is usually required because the infection is so bad, or the symptoms are so extreme, that it can no longer be managed at home.

Many times the hospitalization occurs because the patient has fallen or they are experiencing a lot of confusion, and that is the reason that the family has brought them in. The UTI is discovered after the fact.

In younger people, the traditional symptoms of a UTI are burning or pain with urination, or frequently feeling like you need to pee, but then not being able to go once you get to the commode. For people over the age of 65, this is not always the case. Many of my patients only have the symptoms of a sudden increase in weakness in their legs, causing falling, or a change in their mental status, such as new confusion or a large increase in confusion.

If your older loved one typically doesn't fall and then falls three times in two days, call their PCP or take them to urgent care to be tested for a UTI. If they are normally sharp as a tack mentally, and they are now acting like they can't remember basic information, call their PCP or take them to urgent care to get tested for a UTI. If they have dementia of any type, and are usually a little bit forgetful or confused, and suddenly seem like they are in late stages of dementia and can barely talk to you or answer questions, take them to urgent care to get tested for a UTI!

Dementia worsens gradually. It does not worsen significantly overnight. If your loved one has any type of dementia, and has a sudden large change in their mental status, this is not normal and should be investigated.

If a person has been given antibiotics for a UTI, and they took every pill as instructed, the infection is not necessarily gone. In a younger person, it's safe to assume that one round of antibiotics has totally cleared up a UTI.

In a person over the age of 65, the chances that their body is resistant to the antibiotic, or that the antibiotic was not strong enough to completely knock out the infection, is much higher. Just because they are feeling better, it does not mean that the infection is totally gone. The only way to know that the infection is totally gone is to get tested for it again.

If they do not get tested again, and the infection was only weakened, it will come back stronger and more resistant to the medication. Have the person take all of the medication as prescribed. Wait about 48 hours, and have them tested again. If the infection is still present, they can be prescribed something else while the numbers are low and the infection is easier to finish clearing up.

If the infection is still there but goes undetected because no follow-up testing was done, they may end up having all of the same problems again, including ending up back in the hospital, 10 days to two weeks later.

If your loved one gets frequent UTIs, this should not be ignored. There could be something going on that is creating an environment where they are very prone to this type of infection.

Here are some things to consider:

- If they wear underwear liners or adult briefs, these may need to be changed more often. Urine that is held up against the body creates a breeding ground for infection.

- The same idea applies to any sheets they may be laying on or any sort of towel or barrier they have put under themselves in their favorite chair or in their bed because of incontinence. If they are wet or dirty, they need to be changed.

- Any body fluid around the bottom, including sweat, can also create an ideal environment for infections. If your loved one is prone to sweating, especially around their bottom, they may need to change their clothes more often, clean their bottom area more often, change how many blankets or coverings they are using that may increase sweating, and/or change their underwear or pants to more breathable materials.

- I have seen many patients end up with recurring UTIs because they are not able to take showers anymore, so they are bathing themselves off in the sink. They are either not cleaning their bottoms, or they are using some sort of soap that is not getting fully rinsed off. Changing soap or being more thorough with rinsing after cleaning in this way can help.

- If a person has diabetes, keeping a lot of sugar in their diet can also increase their likelihood of getting to a UTI. Cutting down on sugar in the diet and managing blood sugar levels can sometimes help.

- Staying dehydrated can also lead to frequent UTIs. The bladder is not emptying often enough to keep the fluid (and any bacteria that has come in) moving through the system. Staying well-hydrated can help.

- Cranberry juice or supplements can help prevent or manage the frequency of UTIs. It will not get rid of an infection that is already present, but it can be a good supplement to help if someone is prone to UTIs.

- With women, especially, make sure the person is wiping their bottom from front to back after using the bathroom. If any amount of poop gets wiped forward across the person's opening for where they pee, that can travel up the urinary tract and create an infection. It's very important to wipe from front to back to prevent this from happening.

- Some patients are no longer able to wipe their bottoms the way they could when they were younger due to their size, weakness, or range of motion limitations of their shoulder. If this is true for your loved one, it might be worth getting some occupational therapy for them to help problem solve this issue.

- If you have gone through this list, and nothing is working, make sure and have a conversation with their primary doctor about options. You might want to request a referral to a urologist. Some patients end up on an antibiotic all the time to keep them from having UTIs because they get them so often. This is a last resort and has the added complication of the person building up a tolerance to antibiotics, but if the person is frequently ending up in the hospital over this, it may be necessary.

If your loved one gets UTIs often, and you are tired of dragging them to a doctor's office every time they have the slightest symptom, you can buy over-the-counter testing kits for testing urine at home. This does not replace being seen by the doctor, but if you want to feel more confident that it's worth the trip, doing an at home test that indicates a problem can make it easier to justify making the appointment and taking the time to go to it. This can be especially helpful if your loved one is resistant to going to the doctor and insists that they are fine.

You can find these kits at most local pharmacies or search for them online. If you'd like my recommendation, you can find it on my website at www.helpthecaregiver.com/store.

Summary

Keeping your loved one out of the hospital can take a lot of work. I hope this chapter has given you a lot of good information to feel more confident in helping you care for them when they are sick or hurting.

Again, I can't cover every single possible scenario in this one book, so please join my Facebook page facebook.com/groups/caregiversofaginglovedones or subscribe to my YouTube channel youtube.com/@helpthecaregiverfor more education, information, and support!

Dizziness and falls are a huge problem for the aging population, and can lead to complications that can result in hospitalization. There is so much information in the next two chapters to help you with these issues if your loved one is experiencing them. Please make sure to read through them because there is likely something in there that will be useful to you and your loved one.

Now You Know:

- The major conditions that can cause someone to need to go to the hospital

- How to help your loved one manage some of the major medical conditions they may have

- How to clarify post-surgical instructions with the surgeon

- How to help your loved one manage any pain they may be having

- How to care for a new surgical wound to minimize chance of infection

- How to identify major signs of infection and what to do if you suspect a problem

- How to minimize chance of blood clot after surgery, how to clarify instructions from the surgeon, and what to do if you suspect a blood clot

- Major signs/symptoms of UTI, what to do if your loved one has a UTI, and what to do if your loved one seems to get UTIs a lot

Checklist:

___ You've read the information on your loved one's medical conditions

___ You have asked any questions to better understand your loved one's medical conditions

___ You understand any surgical precautions that apply to your your loved one

__ You understand exactly how your loved one should be taking their blood thinners (if any)

__ You understand how to care for any surgical wounds and know what to do if you suspect a problem

__ You understand how pain management and medication needs might look for your loved one based on the specific surgery they have had (if any)

Notes:

#6 Dizziness

Dizziness is a common symptom that patients often complain about in the home health setting. It can be either a longstanding issue or a new problem for them. Experiencing dizziness is not only frustrating but also poses a significant fall risk and may indicate underlying health concerns. While I cannot know your specific situation, I'd like to guide you through my thought process for analyzing dizziness in my patients, helping you understand potential causes and which healthcare professional to contact for help.

Throughout this book, it's important to note that the information provided is not intended to diagnose or replace professional advice from doctors, therapists, or specialists. Its purpose is solely to offer guidance and help you understand your options for seeking help.

When a patient tells me they are experiencing dizziness, my first step is to determine whether it's likely related to blood pressure, vertigo, or medication. Medications and blood pressure issues can be interconnected, with certain medications potentially causing dizziness.

The first question I ask is whether the dizziness feels like 1) the room is spinning and they might fall over or 2) they feel lightheaded or like they might pass out.

If they describe a feeling of the room spinning, I focus on assessing whether vertigo may be the cause.

If the dizziness is not characterized by spinning, I shift my focus to explore potential blood pressure issues. If you believe that your situation is unrelated to vertigo, feel free to skip ahead to the section on blood pressure.

Vertigo

Vertigo is a term many people have heard but don't fully understand from a medical perspective. They recognize it as extreme dizziness accompanied by feelings of spinning or falling, but they're unsure why it happens.

The most common problem associated with vertigo is called Benign Paroxysmal Positional Vertigo (BPPV). There is a test available to diagnose this condition, which involves the patient needing to lay down on their back with their head in different positions.

Note: if your loved one did not lay down for this test, they were NOT appropriately assessed for this condition. Anything they were told about having or not having vertigo is not official without this test unless they went to an ear, nose, and throat doctor (ENT) who put them through a version of this testing that involves specialized goggles.

Here's the catch: While this test or series of tests may seem simple, it requires a highly trained eye and skill set to interpret accurately. And, the test results can be negative despite the person experiencing symptoms, which is why involving a physical therapist or ENT specialist is so important.

Technically speaking, a person is diagnosed with "vertigo" only if one of these tests has a positive result. Other common diagnoses may include Meniere's disease or vestibular weakness that requires attention and treatment but may not be classified as "vertigo." In this section, I'll use the term "vertigo," but keep in mind that I'm referring to individuals who have tested positive for BPPV.

Now, let's jump into a basic overview of what vertigo actually is, as I typically explain it to my patients. Understanding why vertigo happens can help make sense of the available treatment options.

Vertigo is a problem that happens in the inner ear. It involves several semicircular canals that are inside the skull, deeper than the eardrum, and they are extremely small.

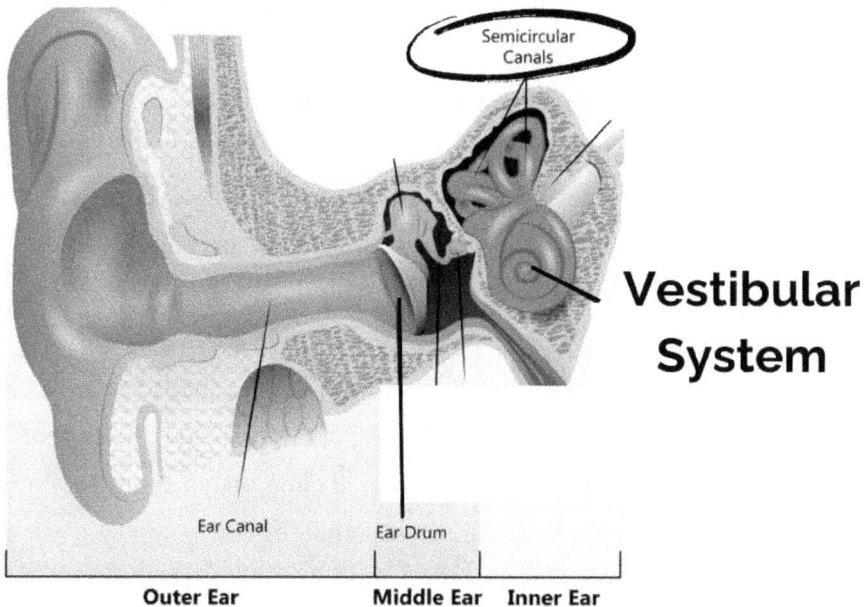

These semicircular canals are filled with fluid and tiny crystals. When you turn your head side to side, up and down, or in any direction, the fluid in these canals whooshes around. As the fluid moves, the crystals hit the canal walls, and the nerves attached to these canals send signals to your brain that tell it about your head's position in space.

For example, when you bend down to pick something up from the floor, this system signals your brain that your head is tilting forward. Even with your eyes closed, you can sense whether you're sitting upright in a recliner or reclining backward. Similarly, in an elevator with no windows, you can still feel if the elevator is moving up or down, partially due to your vestibular system and the movement of fluid and crystals within your semicircular canals.

At times, these crystals can end up in the wrong canal. The exact reasons for this are not always known, but it can happen following a sudden impact, such as a fall or car accident, or after an illness, such as a severe cold that causes pressure changes in the inner ear. Sometimes, the cause is never identified.

When the crystals end up in the wrong canal, they send incorrect signals to the brain. This confuses the brain and can create a sense of falling even when the person is sitting still in their favorite chair. One small turn of the head to the right can cause a person to feel like they are being thrown to the left. Tilting the head up when reaching to put dishes up into a cabinet can cause the person to feel like they've been thrown backward.

This can easily lead to a fall when standing, but it can also cause a fall even while sitting or lying down. The feeling of falling often causes people to have a strong and uncontrollable reaction, flailing their arms, sometimes so strongly that they end up falling out of a chair or bed.

Many patients describe the sensation as if they were being thrown or pushed. I've observed that older patients who fall and can't tell me why, saying things like, "I have no idea what happened. One minute I was standing, and the next thing I knew, I was on the floor," frequently test positive for vertigo.

The most commonly prescribed medication for vestibular dizziness is meclizine, which minimizes or gets rid of vertigo symptoms. However, it's important to note that meclizine only masks the symptoms without addressing the underlying issue. Said another way: it doesn't actually fix the problem!

Here's the good news: physical therapists can help. Let me offer an analogy to help you understand the process. Have you ever played with one of those small tin bb ball puzzles? They were circular containers with clear lids and a picture at the bottom, with perfectly sized holes for one or more bb balls. You had to move the tin back and forth and around in circles to guide the balls to drop exactly into the holes and stay in place.

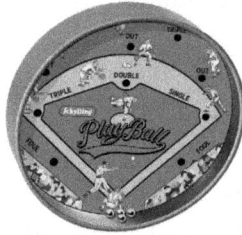

Correcting vertigo as a physical therapist follows a similar idea, but it's not random or guesswork. We use specific head movements to help "drop the crystals" back into the correct canal and make sure they stay in place.

Now, I've come across videos and heard of a few doctors who encourage individuals to "correct vertigo at home." Personally, I strongly discourage this for two reasons. First, there are other conditions related to spinning and dizziness that fall within the same realm as what people commonly refer to as vertigo but are not the same thing. Only qualified professionals, such as physical therapists or ENT specialists, can accurately assess and differentiate these conditions. Additionally, more serious underlying issues may require referral to different specialists, and it would be impossible for individuals to identify or evaluate these on their own.

Second, the process of correcting vertigo can often cause extreme dizziness or nausea. This is a big safety concern when individuals attempt the maneuver themselves or unqualified family members try to help. Falling and becoming injured become real risks in these scenarios.

Let me share a joke that emphasizes the importance of expertise in addressing this problem:

Once there was a world-renowned specialist who was called to fix a problem with an expensive machine. He spent a long time asking questions about it. He walked around it, examined all its corners, and even looked underneath it. Finally, he took out a small hammer, struck the machine once, and it started working flawlessly. A few weeks later, the business owner received a bill for $10,000 for the specialist's service.

Infuriated by the cost, the business owner contacted the specialist, demanding an itemized invoice detailing what was done to warrant such a steep charge. A few days later, the business owner received an invoice in the mail, containing just two lines:

- Hitting the machine once with a hammer: $1
- Knowing where to hit the machine: $9,999

Videos on the internet and downloadable handouts may make the process seem overly simple. While the solution often involves a straightforward series of movements, it is incredibly important to have a professional who has exact knowledge of which series of movements, in what order, and for what purpose, as well as the ability to recognize when specialized referrals are necessary.

If you suspect that your loved one is experiencing this problem, please ask their primary care physician for a referral to a physical therapist, either in an outpatient or home health setting.

One final note on vertigo: Just because a patient undergoes a corrective maneuver to "fix their vertigo," it does not mean that everything will return to normal immediately, or that they don't need any more training or help.

In cases where a person experiences this problem for the first time and gets help shortly after it starts, they may not need much follow-up. However, many of my patients have been suffering with spinning and dizziness for months or even longer before getting help. **Having this problem for a long time leads to long-term side effects that affect balance and stability.**

Here's an analogy I use with my patients: Imagine a healthy, strong high school football player. During a game, a tackle goes wrong, resulting in a broken leg. The player ends up wearing a cast on the leg for approximately 12 weeks.

At the end of those 12 weeks, the doctor may take an X-ray to confirm that the bone has healed and the cast can be removed. However, the player isn't immediately ready to return to the game simply because the bone is no longer broken. When the cast comes off, you'll notice a visible size difference between their right and left legs. The leg that had the cast will be much smaller due to muscle loss from lack of use during the 12 weeks. As a result of this difference and the remaining instability from the freshly healed bone, the player will require comprehensive training to strengthen the leg before safely returning to sport.

The same principle applies to your balance system. If this problem goes on for an extended period, the entire system weakens. Even if the crystals have been repositioned correctly, technically resolving the vertigo, there may still be an underlying balance problem that requires strengthening. Otherwise, issues with balance and stability will continue.

The reason I want to emphasize all of this is to highlight the importance of balance training for individuals who have been dealing with vertigo for a long time. Seeking the expertise of a physical therapist is important, not only for correcting the vertigo problem but also for follow-up care to help the person regain balance and stability, reducing their risk of falls.

Sometimes a person's vestibular system can be weakened just by aging. You know, the old "use it or lose it." In cases where a person has vestibular weakness, they may have similar symptoms to someone with vertigo, but test negative for it. However, they may still benefit from vestibular training through physical therapy.

So what should you do if you suspect your loved one might have vestibular problems? The first step is to call their primary care doctor and request a referral to physical therapy. Some doctors may prefer to refer them to an ear, nose, and throat (ENT) specialist first to rule out any more serious conditions, while others may opt for physical therapy as the first step.

Physical therapists are trained to perform specialized testing that can help determine the need for an ENT referral, and they can help to get that referral from your doctor if necessary. ENTs are more than capable of writing physical therapy referrals. Either way, your loved one will get to the right person that they need to address their problem.

Dizziness Related to Blood Pressure

If an individual often feels dizzy but describes the sensation as feeling like they might pass out, black out, or experience faintness, it's important to consider their blood pressure as a possible contributing factor or cause of the problem.

Low blood pressure can often lead to these feelings, and in extreme cases, very high blood pressure can also be a culprit. In either case, the next step is to check the person's blood pressure. Checking blood pressure every day (at the same time of day) is ideal because it will help you to notice patterns over time or to recognize an unusual reading right away.

If their blood pressure falls outside the normal range, I encourage you to contact their doctor and report the issue. By this point, you should have completed the medication chapter of this book and have an accurate and up-to-date list of all the medications your loved one is taking. This information will be very important to share with the doctor, especially if there have been changes to blood pressure medication during their hospitalization.

If the doctor has been treating your loved one for a long time, they may feel comfortable making immediate changes to their medication. However, if the doctor is less familiar with your loved one's case, they will likely be more cautious about changing medication and may ask you to monitor their blood pressure for a week or two before scheduling a follow-up appointment.

How can you determine if the blood pressure is out of range? I will provide a standard blood pressure reference range here, but I highly recommend discussing the target range with your loved one's cardiologist or primary care doctor. There may be specific reasons why the doctor feels that a different target range is more appropriate for your loved one, but you won't know unless you ask. For more information, and to organize your loved one's vital sign readings and reference ranges from their doctors, consider getting a copy of my Vital Signs log book at helpthecaregiver.com/store.

Blood Pressure Category	Top Number (Systolic)	Bottom Number (Diastolic)	What to do? (Always check that blood pressure meds have been taken.)
Dangerously High	180+	110+	Call 911 or report to emergency room immediately.
Too High	160-179	100-109	Call PCP or Cardiologist for instructions. If no answer or call back. call 911.
High	140-159	85-99	Call PCP or cardiologist for instructions. Set up an appointment to come in. Watch stress and diet.
Normal	90-139	60-84	Good job!
Too Low	80-89	50-59	Call PCP or cardiologist for instructions. Set up an appointment to come in. Watch for signs of dehydration.
Dangerously Low	Less than 80	Less than 50	Call 911 or report to emergency room immediately.

Another way blood pressure can contribute to feelings of dizziness is through a condition called "orthostatic hypotension," which refers to a significant drop in blood pressure when a person stands up or changes positions from lying down flat to sitting up.

For some individuals, this can occur temporarily after a long and challenging hospital stay. They become weak, and experience significant muscle loss during their illness, resulting in reduced muscle support for circulation. As a result, their blood pressure "bottoms out" when they stand up, as gravity causes blood to rush down to their feet, but their body can't effectively return it to their heart and head fast enough.

If this condition is a result of a severe or prolonged illness, it will often fix on its own as the person regains their strength and returns to good health. However, it's important to be aware that this can still be dangerous, because it may lead to fainting or falling. Typically, medication is not prescribed in this case since it is expected to improve on its own. Staying well hydrated and taking enough time when changing positions can help. If your loved one is taking physical therapy, make sure they do their exercises! Strengthening the muscles helps support good circulation and will help this problem pass more quickly.

However, if an individual has been dealing with orthostatic hypotension for a long time, specific medications can be prescribed to limit the drop in blood pressure when changing positions. This may be something the doctor writes a prescription for automatically, or it may be a topic you need to ask about and discuss with the doctor.

By definition, a person does not have orthostatic hypotension unless the top number of their blood pressure drops by 20 points or more when changing positions; for example, a sitting blood pressure of 130/68 that drops to 105/66 when the person stands up.

This is a straightforward assessment that most medical professionals can perform. If your loved one experiences strong lightheadedness or feelings of fainting when standing up, don't hesitate to speak up and request a check-up to see if this is the reason for their dizziness.

A person can experience dizziness related to medication when they are taking too many medications to lower their blood pressure. This is something I have helped many patients discover. There could be several reasons why a patient has been overprescribed blood pressure medication. Here are the top reasons I frequently see with my patients in home health.

1. Weight loss: If a patient's blood pressure medication has not been changed recently, but their blood pressure drops to very low levels after a hospitalization, one of the first questions I ask is whether they have recently experienced significant weight loss or if they lost a large amount of weight during their hospital stay.

Losing weight can naturally lower a person's blood pressure. The amount of medication needed to keep healthy blood pressure levels can be heavily influenced by body weight. If a patient has lost 20+ pounds of weight since they were originally prescribed this medication, and their blood pressure is now very low and causing dizziness or near-fainting episodes, I immediately contact the doctor who prescribed the medication. I provide them with detailed information about the patient's symptoms, how much weight they have lost, and which blood pressure medication they are on. I ask for recommendations and I ask if they would like to make changes to the patient's medication.

2. Multiple prescribing doctors: Ideally, only one doctor should be responsible for a person's blood pressure medication. Typically, this role falls to their primary care doctor or cardiologist. Blood pressure is highly sensitive to small changes in medication, and having multiple doctors prescribing blood pressure medication can lead to miscommunication and overmedication.

I often see this issue come up when a hospital doctor starts prescribing (and/or changing) blood pressure medication. I've seen so many patients who were taking three or four different blood pressure medications prescribed by three different doctors, one of whom was the hospital doctor. Either the doctors were unaware of the patient's complete medication list, or the patient did not receive clear instructions to stop taking one medication before starting another. Regardless of the reason, they ended up taking too much medication.

This is why I spent so much time going into detail in the medication chapter on organizing the patient's pre-hospitalization medication list, documenting changes recommended by the hospital, and providing recommendations on follow-up communication with prescribing doctors about existing or new medications.

If the patient was prescribed blood pressure medication in the hospital and is now experiencing very low blood pressure, it is very important to contact the doctor immediately and provide them with a comprehensive list of all the medications the patient is currently taking (including the new medication prescribed by the hospital), as well as the blood pressure readings you have been recording for the patient.

If a patient is receiving blood pressure medication from both a primary care doctor and a cardiologist, I recommend having a conversation with both doctors to determine who will manage the blood pressure medication going forward. Let them know your preference for having a single doctor to make decisions about blood pressure medication to avoid confusion or potential overmedication.

3. Medication timing and dosage: in other cases, the prescribed amount of medication may be technically correct, but the way in which the patient takes the medication could lead to significant fluctuations in blood pressure. When a person is prescribed multiple blood pressure medications, finding an optimal schedule for each medication may require some trial and error.

For example, one patient may need to take two different medications first thing in the morning because their blood pressure gets very high overnight and both medications are needed to bring it down to a normal range. Another patient may experience a sharp drop in blood pressure if they take two medications in the morning because their blood pressure is only slightly elevated when they wake up.

Some patients may require a single pill in the morning to maintain op-timal blood pressure throughout the day, while others may need the same total dosage split between morning and evening. If you're facing stress and confusion regarding your loved one's blood pressure and medication timing, I have included a special Blood Pressure Troubleshooting Guide in my Vital Signs Logbook for Caregivers, available at healthcaregiver.com/store.

Last Thoughts on Dizziness

Many medications can cause dizziness as a side effect, which poses a significant challenge for patients taking multiple medications. If no other cause for your loved one's dizziness can be identified, it would be worthwhile to review their medication with the prescribing doctors to determine if any medications can be stopped or switched to alternatives with fewer side effects.

While it's not always possible to change or stop a medication, it's always worth discussing with the doctor. Dizziness can be a serious concern because it increases the risk of falls and potential injuries.

I have witnessed patients who outright refuse to take certain medications due to frustration with how dizzy they feel when they take them. If this is the case for your loved one, please tell the doctor about their refusal because of this side effect. The doctor may be more willing to find a creative solution to the problem if they know the patient is not taking a medication that they need.

Keep in mind that there may still be other reasons for a person's dizziness (that I have not covered here) that might be related to other health issues. **If your loved one experiences dizziness along with chest pain, nausea, a fluttery feeling in their chest, or any other concerning symptoms, seek immediate medical attention.**

If it is an emergency, call 911. If it isn't an emergency, but you're not sure which doctor to ask about it, start with your loved one's primary care doctor (PCP) or cardiologist.

Now You Know:

- Several different potential causes of dizziness

- What vertigo really is, and why medication alone can't fix it

- How to record blood pressure and report problematic readings

- How to successfully communicate with the doctors about symptoms of dizziness

Checklist:

__ You recognize high and low blood pressure numbers
__ You are regularly recording your loved one's blood pressure
__ You have reported concerning symptoms of dizziness to the right doctor and have asked for any needed referrals to physical therapy or a specialist (ENT or cardiologist)

Notes:

#7 Falls

As a physical therapist with many years of experience in home health, I have encountered a wide variety of reasons why patients may fall at home. Identifying these reasons is important, because falling poses a significant safety hazard and can cause anxiety for both patients and caregivers.

Why Your Loved One is Falling

There are many reasons that a person might fall, several of which we have already covered. Let's review! When a patient tells me that they have experienced a fall or fall frequently, the first thing I do is ask them what caused the fall. They may not be able to tell me why exactly they are falling, but their response will help me know what to ask or check for next.

If they mention feeling dizzy as the reason for the fall, I go through the process that I described in the chapter on dizziness to assess whether they may have a vertigo, a blood pressure, or a medication issue. For more information on dizziness, please refer to that chapter.

If they say that the falls happen because of their feet getting tangled up or because they are tripping over specific furniture in the house, I go through a safety assessment of the area. I look to see whether there are any rugs that need to be removed, grab bars that need to be added, or furniture that should be rearranged. For additional guidance on general home safety and carpets/rugs, please consult the home safety chapter.

On that note, it's important to consider creative solutions for furniture and other items that impact the layout of a room and ease of movement. Sometimes, it's easy to forget that rearranging furniture is an option, especially if a person has lived in the same house for 50 years without any changes. Keep in mind that with the addition of medical equipment, or a decrease in mobility, adjustments may be necessary for safety.

If the patient says that their knee "gives out" and causes them to fall, they might benefit from a physical therapy evaluation and/or an appointment with an orthopedic surgeon.

There could be many reasons that a knee might "give out" that can be effectively addressed by a physical therapist. On the other hand, an orthopedic specialist can order imaging tests and can determine whether surgery is necessary and if the patient is healthy enough for surgery.

Even if a patient ultimately needs a surgery to fix the problem, many insurance companies will want the person to try "conservative treatment options" before approving an expensive surgery. These options could include pain medication, physical therapy, injections, or other options recommended by the surgeon. So, keep in mind that the person may need to go through at least some physical therapy before qualifying for surgery, if that is determined to be the best option.

If you don't already see an orthopedist and you would like to, ask the primary doctor to send a referral to one, and they can then assess whether or not surgery is a good option.

Regarding knee braces; I prefer not to go into a ton of detail about braces here, but I will say that I believe they are often overused. However, in cases where a patient experiences falls due to a knee giving out, I frequently recommend a knee brace with strong side supports to help prevent falls. If you would like to see the knee brace I most commonly recommend in these situations, visit helpthecaregiver.com/store.

If the underlying issue is that the person is supposed to use a walker or cane because of weakness or balance issues, but has mem-

ory problems causing them to frequently forget and walk without support, the first step is to find the walker or cane in the room. More often than not, it has been pushed to the side, folded up, or leaning against a wall where it is not easily noticeable. When someone struggles to remember to use their cane or walker, they are more likely to remember if the item is placed right in front of them.

Positioning the walker or cane directly in front of where they are sitting helps with better visibility and improves the chances of them using it consistently. If necessary, placing a sign on the walker that says, "(person's name), use me when you get up to walk!" can be helpful.

If they tell me they don't know why they are falling, I ask them if they feel dizzy, lightheaded, or experience knee problems. As I've said in other places, if they say something along the lines of, "I don't know! One minute I'm up, and the next thing I know, I'm on the floor," I'll ask more questions to see if vertigo is really the issue. Vertigo can come on without warning and can basically throw an elderly person onto the floor before they realize what has happened.

If they say that none of those things is the problem, I ask about the location of their falls. Is it the bathroom, bedroom, kitchen? If they consistently fall in the same room, I immediately go to that room with them.

If they are able, I ask them to show me the exact spot where they tend to fall. Often, there is a specific location, and I carefully look around the area for loose rugs, the need for grab bars, tight spaces that hinder the use of their walker, or any other potential hazards. By conducting this thorough assessment, I have solved many mysteries surrounding falls. I have seen things you would never think to ask about, such as sunken areas in the floor that perfectly explain why falls happen there. If they mention two separate places as typical falling spots, I investigate both areas.

Having the person walk to that space is incredibly helpful, because it often reveals the source of the problem that might have more to do with their balance or way of getting around. Watching them make their way to the bathroom, for example, might highlight that the hallway carpet is too thick, causing their walker to get caught, leading to falls. There is no substitute for watching their movements in that specific space, which is why I value home health so much. It provides me with unique opportunities to uncover details I wouldn't otherwise see.

If the person suddenly starts falling (for instance multiples times in a day or week when they typically don't fall), they might need to be checked for a urinary tract infection (UTI). This is especially important if there is also new confusion or a sudden increase in confusion.

In individuals over the age of 65, the typical symptoms of frequent urination or burning during urination may not be present. Sometimes, a sudden decrease in leg strength, an increase in confusion or memory loss, or falls that are out of the ordinary are the only indicators of a UTI.

If you suspect that your loved one has a UTI, they need to have a urine test performed by their doctor. Contact their primary care physician, explain the situation, and ask about the necessary steps to get your loved one tested for a UTI. More information about UTIs can be found in the Staying OUT of the Hospital chapter.

A Final Note on Falls

Over the years, I have learned how to ask my patients whether they have fallen in a way that helps me get an accurate answer out of them. While many patients are willing to admit to having fallen, others are resistant to admitting it to themselves or anyone else.

If a person is concerned about others' reactions to their falls, they are more likely to keep it to themselves or deny it altogether. I have seen many instances where children, especially, start telling their parent what they are no longer "allowed" to do after a fall. This can be incredibly stressful for the patient. Many patients have admitted to me that they have fallen but begged me not to tell their family members because they are afraid of being in trouble or having something taken away from them.

According to Medicare guidelines, the technical definition of a fall is when a person unintentionally ends up on a lower surface than where they started (such as landing on a couch or bed instead of the floor), or an instance where they would have fallen if they hadn't caught themselves on furniture or another stable surface. It doesn't have to be a quick event, and the person doesn't have to end up on the floor for it to count as a fall. Sliding down the edge of a couch until reaching the floor or tripping over one's feet and landing against a nearby wall are both considered falls.

I understand that falls can be scary and have serious consequences. However, it's important to approach this problem as a partnership with your loved one rather than reacting out of fear and potentially starting a fight.

When is it appropriate to ask the doctor for a physical therapy referral? It's always ok to request a physical therapy referral whenever you believe it is necessary. Please don't wait until your loved one has fallen to discuss this matter with their doctor.

Reasons for seeking a physical therapy referral can include: general weakness and difficulty performing daily tasks, experiencing falls or near falls, struggling with activities of daily living such as dressing, bathing, or meal preparation due to pain, weakness, or fatigue, and having unsteadiness while walking.

What should you do if your loved one falls? If the fall results in an obvious emergency situation, call 911! If the person is in severe pain, bleeding, appears confused, or says things that don't make sense, call 911 immediately!

If the person is on blood thinners and they have hit their head, call 911 even if they say they feel fine. They could have a brain bleed and not be showing symptoms.

Sometimes it can be hard to know whether to call 911. If the person doesn't seem seriously injured but you are physically unable to help them off the floor, you can call 911 and explain that your loved one has fallen, you are unable to get them up, and you need help. Emergency Medical Services (EMS) will arrive, help the person move to a safe surface such as a chair or bed, check them for signs of injury, and offer to transport them to the hospital if necessary.

If your loved one is stable and comfortably settled in bed or a chair, EMS will leave. It's important to note that if the patient is able to think clearly and make decisions for themselves, they have the right to refuse transportation to the hospital, even if EMS recommends that they go. While this can be frustrating for all parties involved, patients have the right to refuse medical treatment, including in situations like this.

The exception would be if it is determined that the person is not mentally competent due to a head injury, an infection affecting their mental status, or advanced dementia that impairs their decision-making ability. In these cases, EMTs may make the decision to transport them to the hospital if it is considered medically necessary.

It's important to understand that having medical power of attorney does not replace a person's right to make their own medical decisions as long as they are of sound mind, and healthcare professionals are ethically obligated to respect a person's right to make their own decisions.

Now You Know:

- How to go through a step-by-step assessment to help understand why your loved one might be falling

- Which other chapters in this book to refer to based on your findings

- How to follow up with the doctor if needed

Checklist:

__ You've asked your loved one if they feel dizzy when they fall (if yes, refer to, "Dizziness" chapter)

__ You've asked your loved one if they are tripping when they fall (if yes, refer to, "Home Safety" chapter)

__ You've asked your loved one if their knee(s) "give out" when they fall (if yes, consider a knee brace or request a physical therapy referral)

__ If your loved one forgets their cane or walker, you have relocated them and/or added signs to encourage use

__ If your loved one has a sudden change in frequency of falls, consider having them checked for a UTI (more information about UTIs in the, "Staying OUT of the Hospital" chapter)

__ You have a plan for when to call 911 after a fall, versus when to go to urgent care (such as the person hitting their head and being on blood thinners)

Notes:

#8 Dividing Responsibilities

When you are facing bringing a loved one home from the hospital, or any time you find yourself suddenly thrown into a caregiver role, the list of things that need to be decided or taken care of can feel endless and overwhelming.

Although this chapter can't cover every single scenario for every single person, my aim is to cover all of the most important and common issues I see my patients and their families dealing with in this situation. I will give examples of solutions I have seen during my work in home health, but there are as many different ways to figure these things out as there are families. Always do what feels right for you and works best for your family.

You may not need to address everything that I bring up in this chapter. It's all going to depend on your loved one's medical condition and how much they are still able to do for themselves.

Before we jump into the to-do list, I want to give a heartfelt disclaimer: I know that facing all of these changes and needs, along with the medical issues that caused them in the first place, can be really scary. You may be taking on a caregiver role because someone else who was taking care of these things is no longer able.

Watching our loved ones deal with so many medical problems and potentially being so much more helpless than we've ever seen them before can be heartbreaking and can make us very fearful of losing them. It can be scary to consider the possibility that they may not get better or that we won't be able to give them what they need.

If you are already at your limit in your daily life, as far as what you can physically do or how much time you have to give, being forced to take all of this on, despite not having the time, physical ability, or resources to do so, can create other feelings of anger, resentment, frustration, and impatience.

No matter what you are feeling, it is valid. We will talk more about this in the, "Getting the Help You Need," chapter. However, I want to strongly encourage you to try to keep as much perspective on the situation as possible.

This person who needs help is important in your life. They might be the most important person in the world to you, or they might be someone with whom you have a very difficult or strained relationship. Many times, the answer is somewhere in between.

I have had to mediate many difficult conversations between patients and caregivers over the years. So much of the time, it comes down to either a well-meaning caregiver who is so determined to do everything right that they give very little independence to their loved one, or it is a caregiver who is so stressed out by the situation that they are moving at warp speed trying to "deal with everything" as quickly as possible.

Try to keep in mind that the patient is very likely stressed and over-whelmed too. I have definitely met my share of patients who are perfectly happy to be waited on hand and foot, but the vast majority of patients I see are incredibly frustrated, and many times embarrassed, by how much help they need.

They want to remain as independent as possible, sometimes wanting a level of independence that's not safe at the moment. Many of them are terrified that if they allow someone to step in and help, they will never be able to live independently again.

Very few people in this world are okay with someone coming into their personal space, such as their home, and taking over. How upset would you be if someone came into your space and started sorting through your mail, throwing away things that they decide you don't need, rearranging your furniture, and looking in every cabinet and drawer?

What if someone told you that after 40 years of having the same person cut your hair every six weeks exactly the way you like it, that you just have to learn to live with a different hairstylist who is closer because it is more convenient?

How would you feel if someone asked you to hand over your keys to them so that they could make sure that you wouldn't drive your car, even if you were already resolved not to drive it?

How frustrated would you be if every time you stood up to go to the bathroom or get yourself a snack from the kitchen, someone started scolding you for putting yourself at risk for falling?

I just want to give a moment of pause to consider all the different things your loved one is potentially dealing with right now on top of their sickness, injury, or recovery from surgery.

When you are considering all of the following issues that need to be dealt with, do the best you can to involve your loved one in the decision-making process. As much as possible, consider how they would like these things to be handled. And always ask yourself this question: is this something they can or want to do for themselves?

Consider delaying some of the decisions that don't have to be made right away to minimize the stress on you both. Allow them to maintain as much independence as you safely and reasonably can. Be willing to take the extra time to come up with a compromise that works for everybody if at all possible.

And also be aware that things might change. They may want to do something for themselves now and realize a few weeks in that it's too much for them to handle. They might think they want help with something and then realize it's actually more convenient to just take care of it themselves. This is a learning process for everyone, so make a plan, but be open to the plan changing.

For now, you might be in crisis or emergency response mode, so let's put one foot in front of the other and deal with the needs that are in front of you right now.

When it comes to making these decisions, you might be on your own. You might be the spouse or the child of this person, or you might be a dear friend or other family member. You might also have several interested parties who are all attempting to be involved in the situation. Work through these decisions one at a time. I know you can do this, and I'm sorry for all the stress it causes to be in this position. **You're doing a great job.**

Where Will They Stay?

If they are not going to be staying in their own home, it might need to be decided where they will go instead (for now). Considerations here would include how safe the person is to be by themselves during the daytime, during the evening, and during the middle of the night.

How much are they able to do for themselves as far as using the bathroom, fixing and eating meals, taking their medication, and moving around without falling?

Possible levels of need could include:

1. The person staying in their own home with someone to check on them a few times throughout the day.

2. The person being safe enough to take care of their needs during the day but needing someone to stay with them overnight because of safety with middle of the night bathroom breaks.

3. Needing around-the-clock paid or unpaid care.

4. Needing a high level of help throughout the day but being safe enough to be alone overnight because they do not get out of bed until the morning.

Considerations also have to be made for the person or people who are caring for the patient. It may not be that the patient needs a lot of help during the day, but the caregiver can't reasonably get to the loved one's house multiple times a day to check on them, or can't spend all evening every day away from their own home. The loved one may need to stay at the caregiver's house so that the caregiver can take care of ALL of their responsibilities.

Possible solutions that I have seen could include:

1. The person stays in their own home, but different family members stay with them at different times and then go back to their own homes when their "shift" is over.

2. The person stays with one family member during the week and a different family member on the weekend, either due to differences in work schedules or just to give everyone a regular break.

3. The person stays with whichever family member has someone at home around the clock, possibly with older teenagers living in the home who can also help.

Who is Taking Care of Medication and Doctor Visits?

I strongly recommend that this be the same person. These two items go hand-in-hand, and there needs to be one person who is able to keep track of all of this.

It's too easy for there to be confusion about medication, miscommunication about who has called which doctor to find out the answer to certain questions, or overwhelm about which doctor takes care of which problem, if more than one person is tracking all of it.

Whoever is taking on this responsibility needs to make all doctors' appointments, call in all refills to the pharmacy, fill the medication organizer, and ideally go with the patient to these doctors' appointments.

Whether this is being done by one person or whether it has to be split between more than one person, you can use my "Keep Up with Your Loved One's Doctors All in One" logbook for caregivers to help track everything, including instructions from the doctor. Go to helpthecaregiver.com/store to learn more.

How Are the Bills Getting Paid?

Whether the person is staying in their own home or staying with someone new, the bills will keep on coming! Don't let a major problem creep up by letting the mail go unopened.

Even if this is your spouse, you might not be the one who typically pays the bills, and this can create a lot of stress, trying to figure out where your money is and where it's supposed to be going!

The first thing to do if you are having to help with the finances for the first time is to find out how they usually receive their bills.

If everything gets mailed to the house, this will be smooth sailing! Don't get ahead of yourself. Just make sure the mail is getting checked regularly, and pay the bills as they come in. Don't bother trying to track everything down right this minute and pay everything ahead of time. Don't make things harder on yourself than they have to be! Use mail forwarding if you need to so that all the mail goes to the place where the patient is staying and the mail can be properly monitored.

Some people might have their bills come to an email address. This is much less likely with baby boomers or the silent generation, but every once in a while, you find someone who is happy to jump on new technology and use electronic organization. Hopefully, the person has one designated email for these bills to come to, and it will be easiest on you if you can get access to that email and help them monitor it for bill alerts.

It's also possible that they have automatic Bill Pay arranged with their bank. If that's the case, hopefully, they can also give you their bank login details so you can manage it that way.

Please keep in mind that this person will have to authorize you to speak with any of these companies about their finances. As frustrated as you might be with having to take care of all of this, privacy policies are put in place to prevent fraud and abuse. The person on the other end of that customer service line can lose their job or face serious consequences for giving information to you that they are not legally allowed to give.

Please try to remain patient if you are asked to provide documentation to these companies before they will give you account information such as total balance or balance due. Most companies can take a payment from anyone as long as the account number is known, but they will most likely not be able to tell you how much money is due if you don't already know, until you provide an authorization from the account holder or a power of attorney document.

This will roughly be the same process for finding and managing monthly checks and income. Find out where all the income sources are coming from, and how to access them. Are there checks coming in the mail? Is the money direct-deposited into a bank account? Again, you will need authorization from the account holder, or a power of attorney form, to get full access to financial information.

How is the Person Getting to Doctors Appointments and Other Events?

As I said, I would strongly encourage the person who is maintaining all of the medical information to go with the patient to their doctors' appointments so that they can make sure that everything to do with medication is accurate, to make sure that the doctors are being asked all the right questions, and to be able to consistently record information and instructions from the doctors.

However, I do understand that this isn't always possible, especially if this person works full-time and there is someone else who is more easily able to take the patient to these appointments.

My "Keep Up with Your Loved One's Doctors All in One" logbook for caregivers is a fantastic way to coordinate multiple people being involved in this process. Sit down before the appointment and write out all the questions that need to be asked to the doctor, and make sure there is an updated medication list printed and ready with the logbook.

Go over these questions with the person who is going to be taking the patient to the doctor to make sure they understand what you need them to ask. Have them record the answers in the logbook or on a separate paper so that you can transfer the information into it later.

If the patient goes to the doctor alone, but there is concern about their ability to remember the instructions, consider asking the patient to call you when the doctor is in the room so that you can have a conversation with the doctor and/or hear the instructions that are given firsthand.

For other get-togethers or appointments, it might be helpful to enlist other people for this task who may not have a lot of other ways to help. This could be a dear friend of the patient, a younger family member who is able to take them to a hair appointment on a Saturday morning, or maybe a trusted volunteer from a church group or other community resource.

How are Their Daily Living Needs Going to be Met?

Think about personal bathing, eating and meal preparation, house cleaning, laundry, and if the person needs help getting dressed. How will they get their groceries?

These can be great tasks for someone who will not be taking care of some of the major responsibilities of medication, doctor's appointments, and finances, such as a friend, younger family member, or volunteer. These are also things that are easier to hire out in some cases. If you would like a list of some resources for finding someone to hire, or companies that provide these services, check out the resources chapter at the end of the book.

Some of the services that they would normally leave the house to get might be able to come to them instead. Is there a person who cuts hair who could come to the house? Someone who could do their nails in their home? Delivery service for groceries? Delivery service for medication?

See how much you can get off of your own to do list so you can focus on the major tasks that only you can do.

How Will They Stay Safe?

Are they able to get up and unlock and open the door themselves? Can they hear someone knocking at the door? If not, can a lockbox or smart lock be set up for the door so that a code can be given out to trusted people who may need to come into the home. This is much safer than a hidden key. If you'd like to see my recommendation for one, you can find it on my website www.helpthecaregiver.com/store.

Do they live alone and have a high risk for falls? I am a huge fan of fall necklaces with a feature that auto detects a fall and alerts someone, such as an emergency contact or 911, even if they are unconscious or unable to press the alert button. You can see my recommendations for my favorite fall necklaces on the store site of my webpage.

Is there concern about their safety in their home? A camera system can do wonders for monitoring their activity and safety. I have recommendations for these too, at helpthecaregiver.com/store.

Does Someone Need Financial and/or Medical Power of Attorney?

It's very possible that you need to move paperwork decisions and legal protection to the top of your priority list, especially if your loved one is in bad physical or mental condition.

Please keep in mind that a person can only sign a Power of Attorney if they are of sound mind. If they are already unable to make decisions on their own, they must have a guardian appointed by the court, which is a different process. For this reason, getting a Power of Attorney in place can be somewhat time sensitive and is better to put in place sooner rather than later, especially if the person is in the early stages of dementia.

Links with more information about power of attorney and advanced directives can be found in the resources chapter. If you do not already have an attorney to help you with getting these things set up, you can find one by getting a recommendation from someone you trust, or searching for "estate lawyer (your city and state)". They can help you will everything related to end of life wishes.

Please note that "medical power of attorney" and "financial power of attorney" are two separate things (in the United States). Make sure you have what you need!

Who Will be the Backup Person if Someone Gets Sick?

It's a good idea to think about this before it happens to avoid unnecessary stress and frustration. Do you have a friend or neighbor who could pitch in at the last minute if necessary? If it's not financially possible to have regular paid caregivers, do you have one or two that you could call for last minute help only? Again, information about finding paid help can be found in the resources section.

If you have family members that you would like to be more helpful, but they are not currently involved, I have more suggestions for having a conversation with family members in the asking for help chapter, which is next.

Now You Know:

- Which decisions need to be made for a comprehensive approach to covering your loved one's living needs

Checklist:

___ You have decided where your loved one will be staying (for now)

___ You have decided who is managing medication and doctor's appointments

___ You have decided how your loved one's bills are getting paid (for now)

___ You have decided who is taking your loved one to doctor's appointments

___ You have decided who is taking your loved one to other appointments/events

___ You know who is taking care of your loved one's daily needs like dressing, bathing, meal prep, and cleaning

___ You know how your loved one is getting their groceries

___ You have located services that can come to the house for convenience (like hair/nail services, grocery or medication delivery)

___ You have a safety plan in place (door locks, in home cameras, fall necklaces, etc)

___ You have information about medical/financial power of attorney and/or you have conversations scheduled to make these decisions and get the paperwork in place

Notes:

#9 Getting the Help You Need

Caregiving is not easy. It's difficult to fully understand how hard it is until you are the one doing it. If this is a role you're newly taking on, the shock can be enough to completely overwhelm your system. If you have been caregiving for a while, the burnout can be equally exhausting.

We're going to cover two topics in this chapter: taking care of yourself and getting the help you need. I'm going to give you realistic suggestions for both, so please do yourself a favor and take your time going through this important chapter.

I do want to emphasize how necessary it is to understand and respect your limits. It's not realistic for you to work 24 hours a day and never get any rest or sleep. It's not reasonable for you to never have a day off.

Human beings need rest, nourishment, safety, and connection. Caregiving can easily turn into a situation of total self-deprivation and isolation. I do not want that to happen to you, and I also don't want you to experience guilt because you are (surprisingly!) not superhuman.

I will often remind the caregivers of my patients that if this patient was being cared for in a nursing home, there would be three entire shifts of staff who would be helping to care for them. Everyone would have days off. Everyone would work their shift and go home at the end of the day.

They get vacation time. They get sick days. How can you expect yourself to do it all alone and never have time to rest?

That being said, very few people have the financial ability to have the paid help they truly need to create an ideal scenario. In my experience, there are also very few people who have a family structure that is both willing and able to spread the caregiving load evenly among multiple people in the family.

I would like to see the solutions for caregivers change in my lifetime, but as it stands, it is the most typical situation that caregivers work very long hours, and often around the clock, seven days a week.

This is physically, mentally, emotionally, and spiritually exhausting. Let's see what we can do to realistically provide some breathing room and relief for you. After all, if you become hurt or unable to continue caregiving, both you and your loved one are now in an even more difficult situation.

Self Care the Right Way

In my free Facebook group for caregivers, we take the time to acknowledge Self-Care Sunday every week. It's my way of helping to remind caregivers to keep themselves at the top of their own priority list. I know self-care is a phrase that can cause a lot of eye-rolling because there is very little agreement on what it means and how to realistically fit it into your life.

There are a lot of people on the internet who would have you believe that self-care has to consist of week long yoga retreats and spa days. This is not realistic from a financial or time perspective. It's possible to fit something extravagant like this in on a rare special occasion, but I honestly think that it is more important to find simple, small ways to impact your daily life instead.

Let me clarify how I view self-care: self-care is not about what you do, but about the thoughts and feelings that you put into something when you do them. Almost anything can turn into self-care if you truly regard it as an act of loving yourself.

I've seen many angry posters online who say that "a shower is basic hygiene, it's not self-care, and it's patronizing to say otherwise!" I completely disagree.

Let's say you rush into the shower, scrub yourself down as fast as you can while frantically going through a list of everything in your head you need to do when you get out of the shower. You're feeling stressed the entire time because you can only focus on the other things you really need to get to, and the shower isn't very enjoyable. That isn't self-care at all. That is miserable.

On the other hand, let's say you recognize that you are feeling very stressed and you know that freshly washing your hair and using your brand new bubbly body wash will make you feel like a million bucks. You put down your phone that you've been mindlessly scrolling on for the last 20 minutes and decide that you are going to care for your body and provide a relaxing moment for your mind. Now we are approaching the situation with a completely different energy.

Maybe you set up the other people in the house so that they will absolutely not need you for the next 30 minutes or so, you light a good-smelling candle and take your time in the shower. You focus on how much you appreciate your body for getting you through all the things you need to do in a day, for acknowledging the hard work that you've been doing caring for your loved one, and you focus on deep breathing and all the good smells that relax your nervous system. That is 100% self-care.

How about another example? Let's say you're feeling really tired, and you know that a cup of coffee would give you a little more energy to complete the things on your to-do list for the day. Slamming back a shot of espresso on your way out the door will get you the caffeine boost you need, but absolutely is not self-care.

What if instead, you pour a cup of your favorite coffee just the way you like it into your favorite cup or mug. You sit at your kitchen window or on your front porch and enjoy the weather. While you're in the moment, you purposefully pause and think about a memory, a poem, or a piece of music that brings a smile to your face. That will improve your level of caffeination AND your mood. That is definitely self-care.

What if you turn up the radio to drown out a sound that's aggravating you? Not self-care. What if you turn up the radio because there's a song that just came on that brings on a ton of nostalgia and good feelings, and you allow yourself to sing out loud with a big smile on your face? Totally self-care!

Self-care is a mindset shift, and the actions that we take are helping to make that shift. It's not the actions themselves that are self-care. You could spend a whole day at a spa and spend the entire time thinking about everything you needed to do instead that day, while feeling highly impatient with how long all the services are taking; and I still would not classify that as self-care.

Many people can feel highly discouraged because they hear all these messages about how important it is to take time for themselves, but they don't have the time or money to spend on brunch with friends, salon services, or vacations. They get into a depressed and frustrated place because they feel trapped and deprived. I don't want you to feel that way, so please recognize that this way of approaching self care isn't helpful.

Self-care also does not have to take a long time to be effective. As a matter of fact, it's better to take a couple of minutes of self-care every day or a few days a week than a half day of "self-care" once or twice a year. If you have the ability to fit in bigger things, definitely go for it! But I want to focus on helping you brainstorm ideas that you can implement every day.

You can try to set aside a certain time to do your self-care, but you don't have to. Sometimes it can actually add stress to your day to feel like self-care is one more item on your to-do list, or your stress can get really high if you're not able to do your self-care at the time you had decided. Don't turn self-care into a chore! And don't create financial stress for yourself in your enthusiasm to jump in fully with this idea.

Here are some free or extremely low-cost ways to add self-care to your life:

- Spending some time in a favorite part of the house, like the front porch or a big window with a pretty view

- Listening to music that makes you feel good

- Taking a long shower and adding in a few special products like a great smelling body wash or lighting a candle or two

- Taking the time to serve your meal on your good dishes that all match

- Getting a book of poetry, encouraging quotes, or encouraging passages, like a "chicken soup for the soul" type of book, and reading a page without feeling rushed

- Snuggling up with fuzzy socks, a favorite blanket, and a heating pad at the end of the day

- Trying out at-home spa treatments like a hand mask, facemask, or using a heating pad for your neck that's full of rice and essential oils

- Taking a walk to get some fresh air and increase your circulation if you've been sitting a lot

- Window shopping at your favorite boutique store, shopping center, or mall if you have to run an errand out that direction anyway

- Paying a couple of extra dollars for the upgraded treatment at a salon (or barber shop) instead of rushing through the basic service

- Watching a feel-good movie in your comfiest clothes and popping some popcorn or making a cup of herbal tea

- Getting near some water, whether it is a creek, lake, fountain, ocean, stream, waterfall, or a running water pump you put in your garden. Water is nourishing to the soul.

- I have to throw in the classic bubble bath here. Get some of Dr. Teal's bath liquid with your favorite fragrance of essential oils. Pull up a great music playlist on your phone and turn the lights down. Soak those worries away!

As I've already said, self-care is all about the intention. You're doing these things on purpose because you know they will lift your mood. So before you get started with anything on this list (or another activity you like better), make sure and remind yourself of the following:

"I'm going to do (this activity) because it makes me feel relaxed and happy. I'm going to take my time and refuse to feel rushed, because it's important to take time for myself and keep me at the top of my own priority list."

Managing Your Mental Health at Home

Now, mental health often requires the involvement of other people to have a full and long-lasting effect. Whether that is getting help to manage your stress or frustrations, or whether it is plugging into a community in order to feel seen, heard, and supported, humans are not meant to go it alone.

We will talk about getting direct help with your caregiving tasks in a minute, but I am still focused on you as a person for this next section.

As I've already mentioned, it's not fair or reasonable for one person to have the sole responsibility of taking care of someone else without any breaks or help, but the reality is that so many people are put in this position. The result can be depression, anxiety, overwhelm, and so much more.

There may be times, for whatever reason, that you truly have no other option than to do everything yourself. In that case, it is unbelievably important to manage your mental health.

We just covered a lot of self-care options, and those are all wonderful things to use as part of your overall game plan for managing your mental health. **I want to dive a little deeper into some self-care considerations that can help specifically with anxiety and overwhelm.**

- Weighted blankets are amazing for calming down the nervous system. You can get one on Amazon, and they come in various overall weights so that you can purchase one that has the right amount for you.

- Lavender, chamomile, and mint are three of my favorite essential oils for calming anxiety. You can use them in a diffuser, buy candles that have them as the main fragrances, brew and drink tea with these herbs, use room or car spritzers that have them in them, and buy all sorts of skincare products that use them. I personally love Bath and Body Works aromatherapy products, but anything will do!

- Back off on caffeine consumption. Believe me, I love my coffee! But too much caffeine can make a person irritable, foggy-brained, and generally feeling icky. If you feel like you just can't get to a calm place, evaluate how much caffeine you are drinking versus water, and see if there needs to be more balance there.

- Get back to the basics; sleep, nutrition, and hydration are necessary for you to function effectively. If these needs aren't met, it's going to be nearly impossible for you to feel calm and centered. Take baby steps towards healthier habits in whatever way is possible for you at the moment.

- There are so many free and low-cost apps out there that help with anxiety. One of my very favorite apps is the Calm app. It has breathing exercises, relaxing music, guided meditations, daily encouragement, and even celebrities reading you bedtime stories! There is so much to explore and do on this app, and I reach for it frequently when I need something to help with anxiety or stress.

- If you are a person who uses social media, it's important to realize the effect that this could have on you. It's easy to get lost in negativity, comparison, or just general overwhelm at the state of the world. Check in with yourself and ask if your social media habits are creating more stress for you.

- If you want to have a more positive experience with social media, make a conscious effort to find accounts that bring happiness and positivity to you. I like to follow accounts of people growing flowers, farming, homesteading, animals doing funny things, little kids with baby animals, Italian grandmothers making homemade pasta, accounts dedicated to admiring nature, and accounts focusing on bringing good news.

Help with Mental Health

Everything I've mentioned up to this point is something you can do on your own without the involvement of any other people or groups. Sometimes, you need more support than that, so let's go over some resources that can help.

If you have a job, many employers these days have what's called an EAP, or employee assistance program. This program consists of a lot of resources and often provides free counseling. You will not get unlimited counseling sessions with a program like this, but you can usually get a handful of sessions, which is better than none at all.

Taking care of a loved one brings a lot of stress. With a really good counselor, you can get a lot of quality help in a few focused sessions. To learn about your benefit when it comes to an EAP, contact your company's

HR department. If you're not sure how, your direct supervisor should be able to get that information to you.

Many insurance plans will also come with some similar type of program that can help cover mental health and counseling needs. Again, this would not be unlimited, but a few sessions can go a long way. This would be filed under your own insurance plan, not your loved one's, but put in a call to your insurance provider to see if you have benefits related to counseling that you can take advantage of at low or no cost.

If you feel that you might need ongoing counseling, but you are worried that you cannot afford them, there are many options these days that charge on a "sliding scale." This means that the cost of services can be reduced based on income. Take a look online and see if you can find a sliding scale counseling option that would work for you.

If you feel that your anxiety or overwhelm is getting the better of you on a regular basis, or if you are experiencing symptoms of depression, I strongly encourage you to have a conversation with your doctor about this.

Anxiety and Depression

Anxiety and depression can show themselves in different ways for different people. Some common symptoms for anxiety can include having constant, stressful thoughts, shaking from nervousness, realizing that you are frequently holding your breath because you are stressed, or not breathing in a relaxed way. It can show itself as having very little patience, feeling like the worst is about to happen all the time, trouble sleeping because you can't stop thinking about all the things you need to take care of, crying, or yelling over small inconveniences, etc.

Some common symptoms of depression can include feeling either the need to sleep all the time or not being able to ever get good rest, having a difficult time finding the energy to do basic things like keeping yourself clean or getting enough food to eat, losing interest in things that you normally would enjoy doing, or doing things like eating even when you're not hungry because it makes you feel better. You might even be spending hours scrolling on your phone instead of taking care of very important things on your to-do list, or pulling away from friends and family who are trying to help you.

It's absolutely possible to have anxiety and depression at the same time and experience a mix of symptoms from the above lists.

Please don't let yourself suffer. Many people that I speak with feel guilty or frustrated for needing help with these issues. They feel like they should be able to "get over" their stress on their own. It always hurts my heart to hear people hold themselves to this impossible standard. If you need help, that's all there is to it, you just do!

If you are not able to feel better through the self-care, anxiety management, and counseling options we've talked about, I highly encourage you to ask your doctor about medication. Some people are able to manage their medical conditions with diet and exercise, while other people have to have medication to keep their body in a normal range. It's the same with mental health. Some people are able to manage their stress with self-care and counseling. Other people need help from medication.

It doesn't say anything about you as a person if you need medication to get through an especially difficult and stressful period of time. You wouldn't tell a person to just "get over" their diabetes or high cholesterol. Why do we think it's okay to tell someone to get over their anxiety or depression?

I want to share with you that I have had to take medication for both anxiety and depression in my life. I have been through some very stressful events, and some of them were very long-lasting and kept me in a state of overwhelm at an extremely high level over a very long time. When I started taking medication for these issues, I was better able to cope with the difficulties I was experiencing. I was able to think more clearly, make better decisions, and go through my day without the symptoms of anxiety and overwhelm I had been experiencing.

Even after I had made it through the situations that were causing such extreme stress for me, I still had a lot of work to do before I could manage my stress response without help from medication. I have always been very open about sharing this information because I want the people I speak with about these issues to understand that I absolutely know and fully understand what they are dealing with.

I always thought it was funny when I would tell my patients or their caregivers that I took medication for anxiety. They would frequently tell me that they were surprised because I didn't seem like a person who needed anxiety medication. I would always laugh and respond, "that's because the medication works!"

It might be hard for you to have a conversation with your doctor about wanting medication for anxiety or depression. There can be a lot of fear around being judged or told no. There can be a lot of worry that someone will feel that you are being "dramatic" when you say that you feel like you need medication to help you with these difficulties.

Please don't let these fears or worries stop you from getting the help you need. My depression became so severe a few weeks after my first son was born that I was scared to be left alone. I had a friend who came to stay with me every day while my husband went to work because neither of us felt like it was a good idea for me to be alone all day, and despite all of that, I still knew I would have trouble telling my doctor that I thought I might need medication.

I took that friend with me to my six-week postpartum visit, and her only job was to make sure that I told the doctor what was really going on. And do you know what I did? When he asked me how I was doing, I cheerfully told him I was fine, and everything was going well. I thought my friend was going to fall out of her chair.

It was so hard for me to bring myself to say what was really going on, and I nearly let him walk out the door thinking that I was fine. Luckily, I caught the look of terror on my friend's face and shouted "wait!" right as my OB's hand touched the doorknob to leave. I immediately burst into tears and told him how I really felt, and he was so kind and compassionate with me. We worked together and found a medication that gave me exactly what I needed.

I share this story to make sure you understand how much it means to me that you speak up even when it's hard. Take someone with you to help you share your needs and concerns with your doctor if you have to. Write it down on a piece of paper ahead of time and hand it to the doctor if you have to. Do whatever you need to do to let someone know if you are not okay.

If you do take something for anxiety or depression, don't be in a hurry to come off of your medication because you think you should. Like I laughingly told many of my patients, I didn't seem like a person with anxiety because my anxiety medicine was working so well!

Going on these medicines doesn't mean you will need them for the rest of your life. You might just need them to get you through an especially difficult time. Other people might need to keep these as a permanent part of their medication routine, and that is perfectly fine too. It's about what you need, not about struggling with the question of whether you should need medication or not.

If your doctor does not take your concerns about your anxiety or depression seriously, find one who will. Some people, including doctors, have a very hard time understanding the depths of certain mental struggles that they have never personally experienced.

I have been so fortunate to have had very empathetic, understanding, and supportive doctors on my journey. However, I did have a difficult time with one doctor who I saw when I moved to a new area. That doctor felt that medication should only be temporary and that I should be focusing on counseling and therapy to deal with my anxiety. They were not a fan of writing ongoing anxiety and depression medication prescriptions and made me feel like I was doing something wrong by requesting refills for these medications that I had been taking for a few years at that point.

Because of this, and a few other reasons, I found a different doctor in the area whose approach was a much better match for me. This doctor had no problem at all with continuing my prescriptions, and a few years later, when I told him that I didn't feel that I needed them anymore, he was perfectly fine to support me in that decision too.

If your doctor doesn't understand the concerns you are having or doesn't feel that they are valid, that does not mean that it's true. It just means that their approach is not a good match for your needs, and you are well within your right to find someone else who is more aligned.

Boosting Mental Health Through Community

I want to encourage you to find a way to connect with others more. I know this can be extremely difficult, especially when you are caring for someone who has so many needs that you are not able to spend a lot of time away from them.

In an ideal scenario, you would be able to go in person to see people and do things that lift your spirits. Sometimes, the only realistic community that you can plug into is an online community. There can be a lot of safety and true connection that can happen with people you meet online who are on the same journey as you.

This is why I created my free Facebook group for caregivers, so that people could have a safe and protected space for community and support, to ask questions, and share struggles and celebrations. If you would like to plug-in to a free online community made for caregivers just like you, come join us at facebook.com/groups/caregiversofaginglovedones.

When thinking about community groups, the easiest place to start would be to get more involved in a group that you are already a part of but have not been very active in lately. Maybe this is a volunteer group, a local club, or a place of worship. Are there any groups that you can reconnect with at this time?

Sometimes, when you are on this caregiving journey, the way you connect with others has to look different than it did before you became a caregiver. Maybe it is very difficult or nearly impossible for you to get out of the house, so the fun might need to come to you.

Maybe lunch out with a friend might need to turn into lunch at your house. Maybe instead of shopping with your best friend, they come with you while you run errands, and don't discount this! I had a friend one time who was going through an especially busy and crazy period in her life. I told her one day that I missed her so much and I wanted to spend some time with her on the weekend.

She told me she really missed me too, and wished she could hang out, but she had multiple errands she had to run and couldn't take the time away for us to have lunch together. I told her to let me ride along with her while she did her errands. We were able to chat and catch up while she checked things off her to-do list. We had a great time! Sometimes it just takes getting a little creative.

Asking for Help from Others

Speaking of getting creative with friends and getting the support you need, let's talk about getting some real help for you when it comes to the things you need to do as a caregiver.

You might have a lot of people who are asking how they can help you, or you might not. There can be a lot of reasons why you are not having people offer to help you when it feels so obvious to you that you need it.

If you are the type of person who has always been very independent, others can often assume that you don't need help because you always handle everything alone. The thought is basically that you would ask for help if you needed it, and if you aren't asking for it, you must be doing fine.

Some people can also feel awkward about offering to help someone who has not asked for help because they either feel that it is suggesting that they don't think the other person is handling things well enough, or because they feel like doing so would be pushing themselves on someone who doesn't want it. It still plays into the idea that if the person needed help, they would ask for it, but more from a place of worry that the offer to help would be taken the wrong way.

If you are the person who has been turning down help (even when it has been offered), then I want you to reevaluate why you turned it down and how we can go back and fix this.

I have spoken to many caregivers who were at the absolute end of their rope and completely overwhelmed by their circumstances, who still refused help from anyone who offered it. This usually comes from either feeling that they should be capable of doing it all alone (not true), from feeling that they're causing someone else a problem by asking them to help (not true), or because they are so worried that something will be missed or forgotten if they are not the ones doing it themselves, that their anxiety will not let them hand over a task to someone else.

This last reason is very valid for some things. If you are worried about medication getting messed up, personal care not being done right, or your loved one ending up with skin breakdown, bedsores, or pain from being moved the wrong way, then these might be the tasks you want to take care of yourself to make sure that they are done right.

However, please take a deep breath and recognize that the dishes, laundry, grocery shopping, and lawn care do not hold the same risk of catastrophe if done a little differently than you would usually do them.

I don't say this lightly. My boys were 4 months old and 16 months old when I started my three-year doctoral program for physical therapy. It took a village to get us through those three years. We had a nanny who was helping us full-time, my husband was doing a lot of the care in the evenings, and my grandmother was pitching in a lot to help fill in the gaps.

At first, it was hard for me to let go of the towels being folded differently, the dishes being in a different cabinet every time I went to look for them, and the boys' things always being in different drawers, depending on who had taken care of those chores that day.

I had spent the last 16 months being a stay-at-home mom, and I am very much a "everything has a place and everything in its place" kind of person. At first, this spiked my stress because it was taking me extra time to find the things I was looking for, and it was unsettling that my home didn't look the way I was used to because it was being taken care of by a handful of other people.

The real stress here was coming from me not being the person taking care of my children all day, or controlling their environment, coupled with the sleep deprivation of my little one still not sleeping through the night, and my guilt from being away from them all day.

After a few weeks of feeling full of frustration every time I went to look for a certain dish I needed, I took a deep breath and an emotional step back, and made a conscious decision to lean into gratitude instead. I was so unbelievably grateful to have these wonderful and loving people helping to take care of my family and help us to get through this very busy and overwhelming period of time.

I was so grateful that someone else was taking care of the dishes and the laundry, so that I didn't have to. I was so grateful to come home to a tidy house every day, even if the toys were always somewhere different. I was so grateful that my children were being so lovingly cared for by people I trusted to do the job right.

Again, I share my story to let you know that I understand how hard it can be to let other people help you, but I absolutely promise that if you can shift your thoughts around what is happening, it makes all the difference in the world. If someone is offering to help you, please find a way to let them.

What if no one is offering? It might have to do with the reasons I already mentioned: they don't realize you need the help, or they don't want to seem like they are insulting you by suggesting that you need it in the first place.

I have seen so many out-of-town siblings who have come to visit a patient in my care only to be horrified by how much their sister was doing on her own. They truly had no idea how many things the person was doing, and how much stress they were under, and they felt so guilty once they realized the gravity of the situation.

I have also seen family members who are quick to judge or criticize the way a person is taking care of a family member without ever offering to help or being around long enough to realize how difficult it really is. If you know in your heart that you are doing the right thing by your loved one, then that other person's opinion doesn't matter.

How do you ask for help if no one is offering? The best way is to first sit down and really think about what exactly you would like help with. You probably don't want someone who knows nothing about medication to be in charge of your loved one's medication, for example.

On the other hand, if you feel very overwhelmed by taking care of medication, and you have a family member or friend who is a healthcare professional, that might be exactly the right job for them.

Make a list of the things that you absolutely need to do yourself. This might be finances, medication, doctors' appointments, or bathing your loved one if they are especially private or shy about being helped with bathing.

Also, identify what is most overwhelming to you. It might be one of the things listed above. If you don't have a lot of experience with finances or medication, see if you know someone who does!

When asking for help, it's best to ask for very specific help. Don't just send out an all-call that "I need help!" Put out an all-call that you need help with staying on top of the laundry, or keeping up with the dishes, or transportation to hair appointments.

If you can be specific about what you need, other people can identify an item on that list that they can, or would like to, help with and will be more likely to offer their help.

For instance, I have an incredibly busy schedule that is not predictable. It would create a lot of stress for me to volunteer to take someone to a weekly hair appointment at noon on Fridays. However, I could much more easily swing by your house to do a load of laundry in the random pockets of time that might pop up throughout my week.

For someone else who might have health issues or back trouble, doing housework might not be something they can reasonably help with, but they are perfectly safe to drive a car, and would love an excuse to leave the house to take your loved one to an appointment.

The more specific you could be about the help you need, the more likely you will be to get it.

I have seen every different version of family dynamics possible in my work in home health. Many caregivers are the only child of an aging parent, or they might be one of many siblings and still have all of the responsibility of caregiving put on them.

Some caregivers are the spouse of the loved one who is sick and may have no children who can help, or may have multiple children that they are estranged from who are not involved. These situations can really highlight difficult or dysfunctional family dynamics. It can create an increase in fighting, estrangement, and add another layer of stress to the pile.

If you would like to see a family member helping more, I would suggest that you refrain from accusing them of not caring, abandoning you, making comments about their personal character, or bringing up past grievances. None of this will get you the outcome you are looking for.

However, many times the assumption is that the person taking care of the loved one is handling it just fine by themselves. Reach out in person or with a phone call to explain that you are stressed and overwhelmed and need help. Again, try to be specific about the help you need. Simply saying you need help makes it harder to create real solutions.

If the person doesn't understand the level of involvement of the care you are giving, you might have them take care of the loved one for a weekend so that they can see for themselves how much is really involved. Sometimes it just takes experiencing it for yourself before you can truly understand the gravity of caregiving.

I will say that family dynamics are often complicated, and the stress of caregiving only highlights the difficulties that exist. You cannot force someone to help who is determined not to, so express your needs and ask, but realize that another solution may be needed.

Please also realize that you have the right to put boundaries around the way you are being treated throughout all of this. It is not okay for a person to be treated poorly by those they are caring for or by other family members.

Name-calling, yelling, physical aggression, and intimidation are all unacceptable, no matter how much stress a person is under or how frustrated they are. Please protect your physical safety and mental health from those who are only making the situation harder on you and contributing nothing towards a solution.

If family is not an option for getting the help you need, focus on friends and your community. Communicate clearly what you need, and be sure to ask others to help connect you with resources they know of that can help. You never know who can give you the perfect local referral!

Let's talk about other community resources that might be able to provide some relief for you. Instead of having a paid caregiver come to the house, there may be programs in your local area that can help balance some of yours and your loved one's needs.

There could be programming at a local senior center or community center where your loved one could spend a little bit of time while you run an errand or two. These types of opportunities are great because they give your loved one a reason to get dressed, leave the house, have a change of scenery, socialize with others, and get some extra movement in their day.

It can also be great for you because it gives you a little bit of a break and allows you to complete some tasks on your to-do list without the other person in tow or being left home alone. To look further into community resource options, check out the resources chapter.

Now You Know:

- What self care really is, and how to add realistic self care into your regular routine

- Ways you can address anxiety and stress at home

- Resources that may be available to help with formal mental health management

- Some ways to identify anxiety and/or depression and how to have a conversation with your doctor if you need help

- How to plug into community to help manage the stress that comes with caregiving

- How to ask for help from others in a way that is most likely to be effective

Checklist:

___ You have identified 2-3 free or inexpensive ways to add more self-care to your life

___ You have taken some time to reflect on your current mental/emotional state and you are being honest with yourself about how well YOUR needs are currently being met

___ If you are employed, you have reached out to ask about your company's Employee Assistance Program to see if there are any resources for you that you could use

___ You have identified 1 way you can plug into community more (come join our FB group if nothing else!)

___ You have taken some time to reflect on the potential benefits of counseling and started looking at counseling options if this feels good to you right now

___ You have made a decision about if/when you need to speak with your doctor about help for anxiety or depression if needed

___ You have made a list of specific things you need help with related to caregiving duties, and you are willing to ask for help

___ YOU REMIND YOURSELF ON A DAILY BASIS THAT YOU ARE HUMAN, YOU HAVE LIMITS, YOU ARE DOING YOUR BEST, AND YOU SHOULD BE SO PROUD OF YOURSELF!

Notes:

#10 Resources

Resources are arranged by where they were referred from throughout the book. This is not a comprehensive list of resources, but should give you plenty of starting options. Keep in mind that many recommendations for products mentioned throughout the book can be found at www.helpthecaregiver.com/store. If you are reading this book in a digital format, all the links are clickable.

Introduction:
- Master Checklist download: https://www.helpthecaregiver.com/home-from-the-hospital-checklist

Following Up with Doctors:
- Vital Signs and MD Organization log books: https://helpthecaregiver.com/store

- Keep Up with Your Loved One's Vital Signs (Amazon): https://www.amazon.com/dp/B0CH2D1DHG

- Track Your Loved One's Doctors All in One (Amazon): https://www.amazon.com/dp/B0CH2P1KJR

- Information on palliative and hospice care services: https://www.nia.nih.gov/health/what-are-palliative-care-and-hospice-care

Organizing Medication:

- Medication List download: https://www.helpthecaregiver.com/medication-list

- Organizing Medications download: https://www.helpthecaregiver.com/medication-organization

- Find local drug disposal location: https://safe.pharmacy/drug-disposal/

- Help with paying for medication: https://www.medicare.gov/drug-coverage-part-d/costs-for-medicare-drug-coverage/costs-in-the-coverage-gap/5-ways-to-get-help-with-prescription-costs

Home Safety

- Easy to understand ramp building guidelines: https://upsideinnovations.com/ada-ramp-requirements/

- Oxygen safety instructions and resources: https://www.lung.org/lung-health-diseases/lung-procedures-and-tests/oxygen-therapy/using-oxygen-safely

- Information about Telehealth: https://telehealth.hhs.gov/patients/understanding-telehealth

- Finding help getting to doctors appointments: https://www.patientsrising.org/how-to-find-patient-transportation-services/

Getting Equipment & Supplies:
- Finding insurance for your loved one: https://www.healthcare.gov/

- Help paying for medical equipment: https://nonprofitpoint.com/charities-that-help-with-medical-equipment/

- Directory of US diaper banks by state: https://simonfoundation.org/resources/directory-us-diaper-banks/

Dividing Responsibilities
- Mail forwarding by the postal service: https://www.usps.com/manage/forward.htm

- Information about Power of Attorney: https://www.ncoa.org/adviser/estate-planning/power-of-attorney/

- Create an advanced directive for free: https://www.prepareforyourcare.org

- Private pay help at home: https://www.care.com

- In home service company: https://www.rightathome.net/

- Getting paid to be your loved one's caregiver: https://www.payingforseniorcare.com/paid-caregiver/cash-and-counseling-program#title8

- Home care benefits by state: https://www.payingforseniorcare.com/medicaid-waivers/home-care

Getting the Help You Need

- Calm app: https://www.calm.com/

- Online counseling: https://www.betterhelp.com/

- FREE Facebook group: https://www.facebook.com/groups/car egiversofaginglovedones

- Area Agency on Aging: https://eldercare.acl.gov/Public/About /Aging_Network/AAA.aspx

- Adult daycare programs: https://www.caring.com/senior-living /adult-day-care/

Home Modification Programs (these descriptions and resources found on programsforelderly.com. More resources are available on their website):

- Habitat for Humanity - provides subsidized critical home repairs and modifications for seniors to allow them to age in place and for those with disability or low income circumstances. A "Brush with Kindness" Program for exterior home beautification and the "Repair Corps for Veterans" Program is also featured. http://www.programsforelderly.com/housing-habitat-fo r-humanity-critical-care.php

- Weatherization Assistance Program - Federal program providing weatherization assistance to homeowners with the result of lower energy bills and energy use. US Department of Energy. http://www.programsforelderly.com/housing-weatherization-as sistance-program.php

- Rebuilding Together Safe at Home Modification & Repair Program – Provides critical free home repairs, home modifications and home improvements for low-income seniors, adults and family homeowners. http://www.programsforelderly.com/housing -rebuilding-together-home-modification.php

- Certified Aging in Place Specialist Program – Seniors who plan to stay in their homes as they age can call on a team of trusted aging in place specialists in construction, architecture, and interior design who are available to provide seniors with needed aging-in-place home modifications such as ramps to ensure ease of mobility and elderly home safety. http://www.programsforelderly.com/housi ng-certified-aging-in-place-specialist.php

Notes:

Final Thoughts

I hope that this book has provided you with much needed explanations, resources, encouragement, and a sense of confidence in your ability to carry out your caregiving role.

Please remember that no on can be expected to do anything 24/7, much less care for another person. You need help and support. Use the resources chapter to help you find formal help that can lighten your burden, but don't forget about the personal connections that you need, too.

Sometimes just having someone to vent your stress to, someone to acknowledge how much you're doing, or having someone cheer you on in your victories can make all the difference.

Plug into friends, family, real and online communities. Your mental health is SO important.

Speak up when you have questions or feel overwhelmed, and take breaks when you need them.

Sprinkle in some self care whenever you can, and always with the intention to show yourself some deep care and appreciation for all that you are doing.

Know that I am cheering you on every step of the way. You CAN do this. You're doing such a great job already! Go through the book one piece at a time, check things off the list one at a time. Everything you need to get started is right here, and there are more resources and people waiting to cheer you on in my communities.

Sending all my love and wishes for the best for you AND your loved one!

Master Checklist

Here is a compilation of all of the checklists throughout the entire book. If you would like a digital copy, you can get yours at: https://www.helpthecaregiver.com/home-from-the-hospital-checklist

#1 Following Up with the Doctors:

__ Identify your loved one's PCP

__ Locate any appointments that the hospital made for follow up after discharge

__ Call to reschedule any appointments that were made that need to be changed

__ Call new doctor's office(s) to clarify reason for referral, if you need to

__ Research and decide which new specialists you would like a referral for, if necessary

__ Make a note on appointment to-do list to ask for new referral(s) that are needed

__ Schedule any follow ups with specialists your loved one already sees that have not already been scheduled

__ Decide how you will track vital signs

__ Decide how you will organize MD and visit information

#2 Organizing Medication

__ You have completed a thorough assessment of all the medications that were in the home prior to hospitalization

__ You know which prescriptions are current, and which bottles need to be disposed of

__ You have a list of doctors that need to be followed up with regarding medication questions, including questions about medication your loved one was taking incorrectly, medication they were refusing to take, and new/changed/stopped medication from the hospital

__ You have a list of specific questions to ask each doctor at your follow up visit about your loved one's medications

#3 Home Safety

__ You have a list of any basic supplies you need to get

__ You know how your loved one will physically get into the house when they get home

__ You have a plan for making the entrance/exit from the home accessible (if needed)

__ You know which room your loved one will be sleeping in

__ You have a safety plan for sleeping (safe furniture height, safe furniture arrangement)

__ The bathroom is safe (to get into/out of the room, to get on/off the toilet, in/out of the shower)

__ You have a list of safety equipment needed for the bathroom (nightlight, grab bars, elevated toilet seat, etc)

__ You have a plan for stair safety (if needed)

__ You have a plan for oxygen safety (if needed)

__ You have a plan for floor covering safety (if needed)

__ You know how you will get your loved one out of the house for doctor's appointments OR you have an alternate plan (ex. telemedicine) to keep appointments until they are stronger

#4 Getting Equipment & Supplies

__ You have located the patient's insurance card and the customer service number on the back of it

__ You have contacted the patients "personal case manager" through the insurance to let them know about the patient's needs, including medical equipment and supplies (if applicable)

__ You know the name of the DME company that is being used and their contact number

__ You know what equipment has already been ordered and when it should be arriving

__ All the major equipment needs are ordered or have arrived (hospital bed? wheelchair? walker? bedside commode? oxygen equipment?)

__ You have checked for any quarterly allowance benefit the patient might get, and used it to order needed items

__ You have a list of items insurance doesn't cover, but that your loved one needs for safety or convenience (any of the major items that are not "medically necessary," a rollator walker with a seat, grab bars, night lights, personal care items, etc)

__ You know how you are planning to get the items insurance doesn't cover

#5 Staying OUT of the Hospital

__ You've read the information on your loved one's medical conditions

__ You have asked any questions to better understand your loved one's medical conditions

__ You understand any surgical precautions that apply to your your loved one

__ You understand exactly how your loved one should be taking their blood thinners (if any)

__ You understand how to care for any surgical wounds and know what to do if you suspect a problem

__ You understand how pain management and medication needs might look for your loved one based on the specific surgery they have had (if any)

#6 Dizziness

__ You recognize high and low blood pressure numbers

__ You are regularly recording your loved one's blood pressure

__ You have reported concerning symptoms of dizziness to the right doctor and have asked for any needed referrals to physical therapy or a specialist (ENT or cardiologist)

#7 Falls

__ You've asked your loved one if they feel dizzy when they fall (if yes, refer to, "Dizziness" chapter)

__ You've asked your loved one if they are tripping when they fall (if yes, refer to, "Home Safety" chapter)

__ You've asked your loved one if their knee(s) "give out" when they fall (if yes, consider a knee brace or request a physical therapy referral)

__ If your loved one forgets their cane or walker, you have relocated them and/or added signs to encourage use

__ If your loved one has a sudden change in frequency of falls, consider having them checked for a UTI (more information about UTIs in the, "Staying OUT of the Hospital" chapter)

__ You have a plan for when to call 911 after a fall, versus when to go to urgent care

#8 Dividing Responsibilities

__ You have decided where your loved one will be staying (for now)

__ You have decided who is managing medication and doctor's appointments

__ You have decided how your loved one's bills are getting paid (for now)

__ You have decided who is taking your loved one to doctor's appointments

__ You have decided who is taking your loved one to other appointments/events

__ You know who is taking care of your loved one's daily needs like dressing, bathing, meal prep, and cleaning

__ You know how your loved one is getting their groceries

__ You have located services that can come to the house for convenience (like hair/nail services, grocery or medication delivery)

__ You have a safety plan in place (door locks, in home cameras, fall necklaces, etc)

__ You have information about medical/financial power of attorney and/or you have conversations scheduled to make these decisions and get the paperwork in place

#9 Getting the Help You Need

__ You have identified 2-3 free or inexpensive ways to add more self-care to your life

__ You have taken some time to reflect on your current mental/emotional state and you are being honest with yourself about how well YOUR needs are currently being met

__ If you are employed, you have reached out to ask about your company's Employee Assistance Program to see if there are any resources for you that you could use

__ You have identified 1 way you can plug into community more (come join our FB group if nothing else!)

__ You have taken some time to reflect on the potential benefits of counseling and started looking at counseling options if this feels good to you right now

__ You have made a decision about if/when you need to speak with your doctor about help for anxiety or depression if needed

__ You have made a list of specific things you need help with related to caregiving duties, and you are willing to ask for help

__ YOU REMIND YOURSELF ON A DAILY BASIS THAT YOU ARE HUMAN, YOU HAVE LIMITS, YOU ARE DOING YOUR BEST, AND YOU SHOULD BE SO PROUD OF YOURSELF!

Acknowledgements

I have to acknowledge my amazing husband, Raymond, for the many ways he sacrificed and supported me through this project. Everything we accomplish is a team effort, and this book was no exception. I love you so much.

Jenn, how would I write anything without your help? It means the world to me that you are just as dedicated to getting my projects across the finish line as I am, which is incredibly rare to experience in this world. I cannot thank you enough, and I hope you know how much I mean it.

A huge, heartfelt thank you to those with whom I consulted in putting together the information in this book. Your generous gifts of time and willingness to share your knowledge, experience, and resources helped to shape this book into the amazing powerhouse of information that it is. I hope you are excited by how many lives you will touch through your generosity, because I sure am! Beth, Becky, Jenny, Michelle, & Pam.

About the Author

Julie started college as a music performance major playing the french horn, but ultimately pursued becoming a physical therapist to be able to give hands-on care to others. It didn't take long after graduating PT school for Julie to realize the passion she felt for working with the aging population.

It was her many years of working in home health that inspired her to found Help the Caregiver in order to create change for caregivers who she saw doing so much with so little help.

Julie was born and raised in Georgia, where she currently lives with her husband and 3 children.

She loves spending quality time with her family any way that will put her near water, whether it's by the beach, lake, pool, or hiking to a beautiful waterfall.

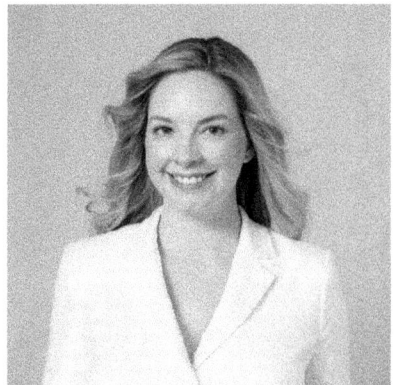

Dr. Julie Crenshaw, PT, DPT

Also By...

Get all 3 books in the Caregiver Support series. Available on Amazon
or www.helpthecaregiver.com/store

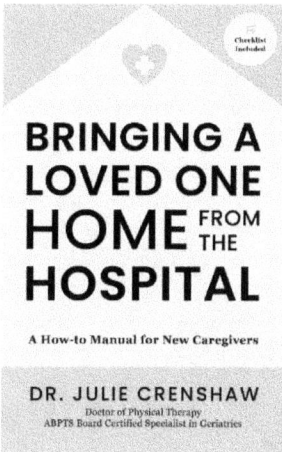

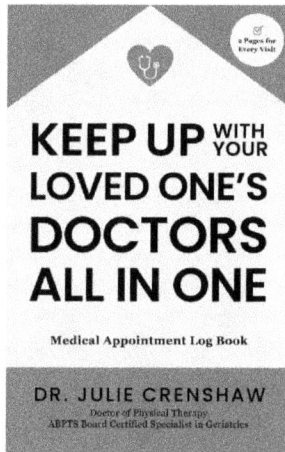

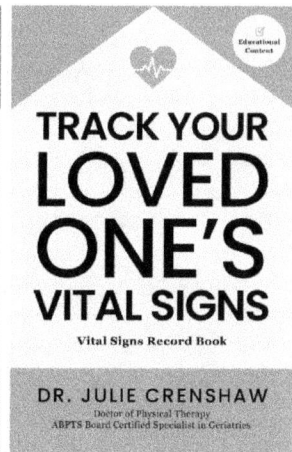

BRINGING A LOVED ONE HOME FROM THE HOSPITAL
A How-to Manual for New Caregivers
DR. JULIE CRENSHAW
Doctor of Physical Therapy
ABPTS Board Certified Specialist in Geriatrics

KEEP UP WITH YOUR LOVED ONE'S DOCTORS ALL IN ONE
Medical Appointment Log Book
DR. JULIE CRENSHAW
Doctor of Physical Therapy
ABPTS Board Certified Specialist in Geriatrics

TRACK YOUR LOVED ONE'S VITAL SIGNS
Vital Signs Record Book
DR. JULIE CRENSHAW
Doctor of Physical Therapy
ABPTS Board Certified Specialist in Geriatrics